Essential Clinical Social Work Series

Series Editor
Carol Tosone, School of Social Work, New York University, New York, NY, USA

The Essential Clinical Social Work Series provides state-of-the-art theoretical and clinical knowledge for clinical social workers and other mental health practitioners.

More information about this series at http://www.springer.com/series/8115

Katherine Compitus

The Human-Animal Bond in Clinical Social Work Practice

Springer

Katherine Compitus
NYU Silver School of Social Work
New York, NY, USA

ISSN 2520-162X ISSN 2520-1611 (electronic)
Essential Clinical Social Work Series
ISBN 978-3-030-87782-8 ISBN 978-3-030-87783-5 (eBook)
https://doi.org/10.1007/978-3-030-87783-5

This Springer imprint is published by the registered company Springer Nature Switzerland AG
The registered company address is: Gewerbestrasse 11, 6330 Cham, Switzerland

This book is dedicated to Morgan, Angie, Eros, and Boston. Although they were not the first animals to touch my heart, nor will they be the last, they taught me that human beings still have so much to learn about the unconditional positive regard and social support that comes so naturally to other animals.

Foreword

A couple weeks prior to this writing, I bid farewell to my remarkable play therapy dog, Kirrie. She was 17.5 years old, and we had lived together from the time she was 9 months. We had worked together for 12 of those years. We shared a reciprocal relationship in which I tried to consider her needs and preferences every step of the way, and she decided whether or not she wanted to be involved in my work at any given moment. She worked off-leash and freely made those choices for herself. She typically was eager to engage with my clients or the mental health professionals in my workshops because she was so sociable, playful, and curious. Clients and colleagues were pleased because she *chose* to work with them, and they appreciated the authenticity of that experience. Just a few weeks prior to her death, her very arthritic legs did not keep her from slowly walking over to the training center to greet the therapists who had come to learn about the work she had inspired. I was fortunate to have a therapy partner who taught me how rich a mutually beneficial relationship between human and animal could be. And how therapeutic that mutually respectful relationship could be for so many.

Interest in Animal-Assisted Interventions (AAIs) has grown dramatically during recent years, and the benefits of the human-animal bond have been increasingly studied from the perspective of many disciplines and applied to many physical and psychosocial challenges for people of all ages. While the benefits for humans have been clearly demonstrated through research and clinical experience, the picture of the impact on the animals is less clear. Only recently have studies, articles, and books begun to explore the critical questions surrounding potential benefits or downsides of AAIs for the animals who are involved. Furthermore, there are still too many who involve animals in their work while remaining unaware of the complexities of AAIs and who fail to obtain sufficient training and supervision, not only in effective clinical practice with animals but also in understanding their animal therapy partners as fully as possible.

With the rapidly growing interest among professionals in the human-animal bond coupled with the lagging awareness of the multiple competencies needed to work effectively and ethically with animals, there is a need for the professional literature to offer theoretical, empirical, applied, and welfare information as this broad field evolves. Dr. Katherine Compitus comes to this task with a combined background in animal behavior, positive animal training, and doctoral-level clinical social work. She operates a private nonprofit sanctuary for many species of animals where she focuses on creating a healing environment for all involved. She has a passion for learning the lessons that animals teach about healing, mindfulness, health, and being more humane humans. In this book, she explores the many facets of the human-animal bond and the multiple ways that humans can work respectfully and compassionately with animals. It explores the many facets of AAIs and how human lives are enriched by getting to know animals on their own terms as the unique and sentient beings they are.

Risë VanFleet, PhD, RPT-S, CDBC, CAEBI
Licensed Psychologist, Registered Play Therapist-Supervisor,
Certified Dog Behavior Consultant, Certified Animal Ethology
and Behavior Instructor
President, International Institute for Animal Assisted Play Therapy®
Author (with Tracie Faa-Thompson), the Maxwell Award-winning
book, *Animal Assisted Play Therapy* (and several other books on play therapy,
Filial Therapy, Animal Assisted Play Therapy®, and animal behavior)
Boiling Springs, PA, USA

Preface

I feel very fortunate that I grew up surrounded by a multitude of pets. As a child I shared my home with fish, gerbils, guinea pigs, rabbits, and cats. In summers at camp, or on weekends with friends, I would get to go horseback riding and play with other species of animals. I had friends with pet iguanas, snakes, and dogs. I always wanted a dog, but I was highly allergic as a child. It wasn't until I was in college that I realized that I had outgrown my allergy and my connection to dogs was able to fully develop. I thought, as a child, that I wanted to be a veterinarian or a marine biologist, but through the twists and turns of life I was drawn to education and clinical social work. Within these fields, however, I found my way back to animals through close study of the human-animal bond (HAB). For over a decade, I have been forging my own path in the social work field applying this study of HAB. Although every day I meet people who are interested in this exciting, innovative, and burgeoning field, there remain so many gaps in knowledge and gaps in service that I have felt compelled to write this book. I hope you will enjoy it; it would take volumes to cover everything I have to say, but I have done my best to distill the most important insights I can offer within these pages. I hope it inspires other clinicians to continue their research, as well as their direct social work, their concrete and clinical services helping people with pets. This book was really written as a gift from the heart, from me to all of you.

New York, NY, USA — Katherine Compitus

Acknowledgments

Although I absolutely love this field, I had a difficult time writing this book in 2020. In the same year I completed my doctorate, I also contracted COVID, had a mild traumatic brain injury, and lost one of my beloved dogs, Boston, suddenly to cancer. I could not have written this book without the continuous support of, and reminders from, my husband, Paul. This book would never have happened without you. I would also like to thank my mentors, including Dr. Carol Tosone, Dr. Risë VanFleet, and Dr. Aminda Heckman, for believing in me as a clinician, an academic, and a writer. I would like to thank Milagros Sanchez-Nester for encouraging me to be not only the person but also the social worker that I always knew I was deep inside. I would also like to thank some of the amazing professors and administrators at New York University (NYU) who pushed me to be my best, challenged me, and nurtured my academic goals. This list includes Dr. Linda Laussell-Bryant, Dr. Jean Anastas, and director Benjamin Sher. I would like to thank Dr. Marc Bekoff for his support of a budding author and fellow animal behaviorist. My friend Melissa Burgos is an expert in working with animal hoarders and taught me a great deal about working with people with pets. I would also like to thank Jennifer Robertson and Marie O'Shea for their assistance with copy-editing.

I would like to thank all my friends and, of course, my family. My parents, Gladys and Norman, and sisters, Alexandra (and her husband Samir) and Jennifer, have an amazing love and respect for animals that runs deep, and we continue to learn from one another. I also must thank Melissa Burgos, who taught me a lot about the world of animal rescue and best practices with animal hoarding situations. Last, but always first in my heart, are all of the animals that I have had the honor of sharing my life with. It is only through my relationship with these amazing and intelligent beings that I learned that we really cannot call ourselves human until we learn how to be humane.

Contents

About the Author

Katherine Compitus DSW, LCSW, MSEd, MA, is a doctor of clinical social work and an anthrozoologist. Her research focuses primarily on social policy, mental health, and the human-animal bond. Katherine is the founder and chairman of Surrey Hills Sanctuary, a non-profit organization providing veterinary social work services to trauma and abuse survivors in New York State. She has lectured extensively on Animal-Assisted Therapy, Grief Counseling for Pet Loss, Suicidality in Veterinary Professionals, and Crisis Intervention for People with Pets. Katherine is currently a lecturer in the graduate social work schools at Columbia University, Fordham University, and New York University (NYU), where she developed and currently teaches the Human-Animal Bond course at NYU's Silver School of Social Work. Early in her social work career Katherine provided bilingual animal-assisted therapy at the NYU Hospital for Joint Diseases, helped establish a therapy animal program at an AHRC preschool, and was a grief counselor for pet loss at the Animal Medical Center in New York City. Born and raised in New York City, she now spends most of her time in upstate New York with her husband and the 40+ animals at the sanctuary, including chickens, potbellied pigs, pigeons, cats, dogs, and two naughty stee (bulls).

Abbreviations

AAA	Animal-Assisted Activity
AACR	Animal-Assisted Crisis Response
AAE	Animal-Assisted Education
AAI	Animal-Assisted Intervention
AAT	Animal-Assisted Therapy
AAPT	Animal Assisted Play Therapy®
ADA	Americans with Disabilities Act
APBT	American Pit Bull Terrier
BAT	Bovine-Assisted Therapy
BPD	Borderline Personality Disorder
DBT	Dialectical Behavior Therapy
DSM-V	The Diagnostic and Statistical Manual of Mental Disorders, 5th Edition
DSRD	Disaster Stress Relief Dog
ET	Equine Therapy
ESA	Emotional Support Animal
HAB	Human-Animal Bond
HABRI	The Human-Animal Bond Research Institute
HARC	Hoarding of Animals Research Consortium
HARP	Human-Animal Relational Processing
NASW	National Association of Social Workers
NIH	National Institutes of Health
PACT	Preventing Animal Cruelty and Torture
PSD	Psychiatric Service Dog
SD	Service Dog
TD	Therapy Dog
TDI	Therapy Dogs International

Chapter 1
Introduction

I have always had an affinity toward animals and felt that my own mood improved when I was around them. My social work career with animals began my first year at New York University. I was an intern at the Hospital for Joint Diseases, working with older, Spanish-speaking adults in the ambulatory care clinic. As they came in to speak to me about concrete services, it often initiated a clinical session. One older woman who was due for knee surgery mentioned that she had a diabetic cat that required insulin shots daily. On a limited income, she reported feeling significant distress that she might not be able to both feed herself and cover the medical supplies for her cat. The woman reported to me that she was estranged from her family and housebound, and saw her cat as a primary source of love and support; she was unable to imagine life without him. After speaking to her about possible resources for her and her cat (there were few at the time), I began to ask more of my clients about the pets in their lives. I discovered that even when a client was reluctant to engage in therapy, they were happy to speak about their pets, both current and past. This helped build a faster rapport, which in turn allowed me to better help them secure the services that they needed. It also led me to think more pointedly about the role that animals and pets play in a person's emotional life.

As I continued in my social work career, I made a point to seek out any experience that I could in animal-assisted therapy (AAT) or work exploring the human–animal bond (HAB). I provided pediatric AAT services to children who had recently undergone surgery, helped create a therapy dog program at a preschool for children with developmental delays, and was fortunate to be one of the last social work interns at the Animal Medical Center (AMC) in New York City before the Center's social work department closed for several years due to budget cuts. During my time in the department we helped provide communication training to veterinarians, supported the veterinary staff to minimize compassion fatigue and burnout, and focused especially on clinical therapy services such as grief counseling for pet loss or support through difficult medical decisions. (The hospital recently reopened the department, but I am still surprised at the lack of clinical social workers in most major

K. Compitus, *The Human-Animal Bond in Clinical Social Work Practice*,
Essential Clinical Social Work Series,
https://doi.org/10.1007/978-3-030-87783-5_1

veterinary hospitals, a gap in service that needs to be addressed.) Throughout my career, I have continued to witness how concrete services have the potential to lead to clinical intervention, and that there is a dire need for both concrete services and clinical social work addressing the human–animal bond.

So, what exactly is the human–animal bond? The American Veterinary Medical Association (AVMA) describes it as "a mutually beneficial and dynamic relationship between people and animals that is influenced by behaviors essential to the health and well-being of both. This includes, among other things, emotional, psychological, and physical interactions of people, animals, and the environment. The veterinarian's role in the human-animal bond is to maximize the potential of this relationship between people and animals" (American Veterinary Medical Association, n.d.). It is important to note that this relationship is dynamic, evolving, and benefits both the human and animal. Chapter 2, covering the history of HAB, will discuss how the potential of animals to improve psychological health has been recognized for hundreds of years, but only fairly recently have scientists and clinicians undertaken formal research into the myriad ways the bond may benefit both people and pets.

To date, most books on HAB address the subject from a purely psychological perspective. This book is different because I attempt to address it also from a social welfare perspective, taking into account the variety of ways in which social workers may help clients find and utilize their own strengths to return them to a state of equilibrium. Social workers practice a type of therapy that uses a strengths-based perspective, which means that we first assess a client's innate and learned skills and talents, and how they may be used to address whatever hardship a client is undergoing. This framework is holistic, taking into account an individual's emotions, experiences, and environment. Social workers help clients make an inventory of their perceived strengths and weaknesses in order to build a series of steps toward positive life changes, building on the strengths or addressing perceived challenges. This approach can be understood through the lens of work by Carl Rogers (1957), who developed the concept of therapists' "unconditional positive regard" toward their clients, and Karen Horney, who discussed the idea of "wholeheartedness" on the part of the therapist as essential to a client's success in therapy (Zalayet, 2020). Although neither was speaking directly about social workers, both approached the therapeutic process from a strengths-based perspective. This is the primary difference between social workers and other mental health professionals, such as psychologists and psychiatrists. Rather than ask "What is wrong with you?" I prefer to ask a client, "What has happened to you?"

This type of framework is ideally suited to clinical work that deals with HAB, since it is an integral part of many people's lives that is routinely undervalued. For example, those who suffer the death of a beloved pet often find themselves alone, misunderstood by a society that tends to regard pet guardianship as superficial. I postulate that HAB is deep, innate, and powerful—a right that all humans deserve to experience, rather than a privilege. In fact, I would go so far as to say HAB is a basic biological need, and it is important for clinicians to remember that a person will struggle to find emotional stability until such needs are met. However, as important as HAB is, it is important for clinicians to consider all aspects of the person-in-environment and ask whether the clients' basic biological needs are first being met; until this condition is satisfied, they will likely struggle to find emotional stability no matter what clinical intervention is offered.

Definitions

Before I delve into the history of HAB, I must first define some of the more common terms used when discussing the topic (I have also included in this book a list of abbreviations to help the reader).

Animal-Assisted Therapy (AAT) describes the integration of an animal into direct clinical practice. *Animal-Assisted Interventions (AAI)* are the integration of an animal into activities that may not involve direct clinical work or be led by a psychotherapist, but still may provide some therapeutic benefit to participants. A *therapy animal* is one which is integrated into direct clinical practice. A *service animal (SA)* is a dog or miniature horse, and works as a tool to aid a person with a physical or psychological disability to navigate their daily activities. An *emotional support animal (ESA)* is an animal that helps someone with mental illness in their attempt to self-soothe.

These last three terms are a source of confusion for many clinicians and laypeople. *A service animal* may go anywhere a person can go, just as a wheelchair would assist a person with limited mobility get around more easily. A service animal must be highly trained to perform certain tasks to aid their disabled handler, and service animals and their handlers are protected from discrimination under the Americans with Disabilities Act (ADA). Although a psychiatric service animal does provide a therapeutic service, their primary task is to help their handler complete their day-to-day activities.

In contrast, a *therapy animal* provides therapeutic services first and foremost, and cannot go into a restaurant or movie theater. Most therapy animals are evaluated and certified by an independent therapy animal agency and are only allowed in places that have contracted with the agency or handler to have supervised visits, such as at a hospital, school, clinic, or private practice. Additionally, a therapy animal usually helps more than one person, while a service animal is trained to assist one select person. The therapy animal's handler may be a psychotherapist/social worker or may be another person, perhaps the animal's guardian (the therapist and handler do not have to be the same person).

There has been a lot of controversy over the rights of people with animals that fall into the last category, emotional support animals. In contrast to the therapy animal, and more similarly to the service animal, an emotional support animal provides assistance to just one person. However, unlike a service animal, an ESA is not covered under the ADA and, therefore, has no special privileges or rights, except for those established by previous laws such as the ability to accompany their guardian in the cabin of an airplane or being allowed in housing which normally does not allow pets. In this regard, ESAs fall somewhere between a service animal, a therapy animal, and a pet, with few of the rights of a service animal but also none of the requirements.

What Do SA, ESA, and Therapy Animals Do?

The types of therapy animals and service animals are too numerous to mention here. Service animals may help people with hearing or vision impairments, or, since other animals have more sensitive olfactory systems than humans, they may help people with chemical sensitivities avoid dangerous areas. They help people with multiple types of mobility issues, or may be psychiatric service dogs, helping veterans with PTSD or those with bipolar disorder. A defining aspect of service dogs is that they perform tasks specific to the needs of the people they serve. A guide dog for a blind person must know how to navigate the streets with their handler. A PTSD psychiatric service dog may sit facing the direction opposite their handler, so the handler feels their back is always protected.

Just as there are numerous types of service dogs, there are many types of therapy dogs. Therapy dogs may be found in hospitals, helping boost the morale of long-term patients or those recovering from surgeries. They can be found in assisted living facilities for older adults. Research shows that therapy animals may help prevent dementia (Friedmann et al., 2019), or in schools, inspiring children with learning disabilities to practice reading out loud (Hall et al., 2016). They may also be on the front lines of national crises, such as school shootings or terrorist attacks, working as crisis response animals, where they may facilitate rapport between social worker and client in order to provide clients with immediate relief from trauma in a time of acute need.

Although more limited in scope, there are many circumstances when the company of an ESA is highly beneficial. If a fear and/or phobia are localized to flying, then an ESA accompanying the client on an airplane may help alleviate that stress. I have seen this type of phobia in clients who lived in New York City during the World Trade Center attacks on September 11. Although a person may not have been near the site when the attacks happened, the secondary and proximal trauma caused by the terrorist attacks affected many people to a degree significant enough for the inclusion of an ESA into their travel plans. I have also seen the benefits of ESAs in easing housing transitions for clients who were previously undomiciled or who are fleeing a dangerous situation, such as one involving intimate partner violence. This will be discussed in depth in a later chapter, but many clients do not want to enter into safe housing without their beloved pet. ESA laws allow for companion animals in buildings that normally do not allow pets. This allows people to maintain the continued (and sometimes only) support system of their pets while reestablishing a state of equilibrium.

It is my position that most interactions with animals have therapeutic benefits and that such benefits take many forms. Unfortunately, the law is generally not well-defined when it comes to any of these types of assistance animals (most notably ESAs), which leaves these categories open to abuse and misuse. If the welfare of the animal is being harmed by defining it as an ESA (e.g., bringing a peacock into an airport is not species-appropriate behavior), then my position is that the animal should never be misused in this way. When the animal is at risk, then the therapeutic possibilities are lost to the person as well (see section on animal welfare).

Chapter Summaries

This is a large and growing field and I could not include every aspect of the human–animal bond in one book; I tried to restrict this book to those topics most relevant to HAB in clinical social work. This book started with definitions of the terms most often used within HAB-related work and clinical psychotherapy. In Chap. 2, I will provide a foundation for HAB in clinical social work by discussing the long history of the relationship between people and animals, the evolution of animal-assisted interventions (AAI), and early interventions by famous historical figures such as Florence Nightingale and Sigmund Freud. In Chap. 3, I examine the biopsychosocial model as a working hypothesis and contextual framework, including a discussion of why the human–animal bond is so powerful, by examining this relationship through a biological perspective, a psychological perspective, and a social perspective. In Chap. 4, I will discuss the process of conducting animal-assisted therapy, including the preparation and assessment, the integration of animal-assisted therapy (AAT) with various treatment models, and therapy animal welfare issues. Chapter 5 includes a further discussion of clinical treatment, specifically as it pertains to veterinary social work, or the intersection of veterinary medicine and social work fields. This includes an exploration of compassion fatigue in the veterinary profession (including the high rate of suicidality in veterinarians) and grief counseling for pet loss. Chapter 6 addresses crisis intervention services in HAB, with a discussion of topics such as homelessness, domestic violence, disaster relief, and the effect of breed-specific legislation. Although these may appear to be purely concrete services, working with people in crisis almost always results in additional clinical interventions. Finally, in Chap. 7, I conclude this book with a discussion of the limitations of and future directions in HAB, including a brief discussion of the clinical nature of animal hoarding.

Conclusion

Hartwig and Smelser (2018) studied practitioner perspectives on animal-assisted psychotherapy in great detail; they found that the vast majority of social work practitioners believe animal-assisted therapy and knowledge of HAB in direct clinical practice would be very useful. However, these same practitioners reported not knowing where to get more information on HAB or how to integrate it into their practice. Although this is a growing field, there are still many gaps in service and many clinicians that are left curious about how to get started in HAB and AAT. I hope this book will pull back the curtain so that clinical social workers and mental health practitioners of all types can start expanding their practice to include pets as an integral part of the human experience.

A Final Note of Caution

Animal interaction in direct clinical practice should always be a mutually beneficial relationship. The animals should never be forced to perform or used as props. Animal welfare, as discussed later in this book, is of the utmost importance and should always be considered in any therapeutic interaction. A basic knowledge of species-appropriate behaviors is, therefore, beneficial to any clinician interested in integrating animals into their clinical practice.

References

American Veterinary Medical Association. (n.d.). *Human–animal bond.* Author. Retrieved from https://www.avma.org/kb/resources/reference/human-animal-bond/pages/human-animal-bond-avma.aspx. [Not cited in chapter; also article not found on AVMA site].

Friedmann, E., Galik, E., Thomas, S. A., Hall, S., Cheon, J., Han, N., Kim, H. J., McAtee, S., & Gee, N. R. (2019). Relationship of behavioral interactions during an animal-assisted intervention in assisted living to health-related outcomes. *Anthrozoös, 32*(2), 221–238.

Hall, S. S., Gee, N. R., & Mills, D. S. (2016). Children reading to dogs: A systematic review of the literature. *PLoS One, 11*(2), e0149759. [Not cited in chapter].

Hartwig, E. K., & Smelser, Q. K. (2018). Practitioner perspectives on animal-assisted counseling. *Journal of Mental Health Counseling, 40*(1), 43–57.

Rogers, C. R. (1957). The necessary and sufficient conditions of therapeutic personality change. *Journal of Consulting Psychology, 21*(2), 95.

Zalayet, J. (2020). Wholeheartedness in the treatment of shared trauma: Special considerations during the COVID-19 pandemic. In *Shared trauma, shared resilience during a pandemic* (pp. 179–185). Springer.

Chapter 2
A Brief History of the Human–Animal Bond

I have already explained the significance of some of the most frequently used terms related to HAB, such as animal-assisted therapy or emotional support animals. Now I will discuss the source of these terms: how HAB started, from scavenging animals bonding with cavemen to math problem-solving horses, from animals integrated into medical treatments through to HAB's current development into a psychotherapeutic treatment model. Although applied anthrozoology (the direct application of HAB) is still a burgeoning field, we have known about the psychological benefits of interacting with other species of animals for quite some time. You may be surprised to recognize quite a few famous names sprinkled throughout this chapter, figures whose therapeutic work with animals is often forgotten.

Historical Foundations of HAB

It makes sense to begin with "man's best friend": Scientists currently believe that dogs were among the first domesticated animals, although exactly how long ago this relationship began is uncertain (Larson et al., 2012). Drawings in the Arabian Peninsula, some dating back 8000 years, depict canines interacting with men (Degerbøl, 1961). These images show dogs hunting in collaboration with men or protecting men from other predatory animals. Some of these dogs are leashed and tethered to the humans, suggesting that they may be younger dogs in training. Notably, despite the age of the drawings, the canines shown appear very dog-like, with pointed ears and curly tails that differentiate them from wolves and hyenas, which were most likely the first domesticated canines (Ostrander et al., 2017). In the scientific community it is speculated, based on such cave drawings and on carbon dating performed on preserved remains of domesticated canines, that the human–dog relationship started approximately 14,000 years ago (some scientists postulate

K. Compitus, *The Human-Animal Bond in Clinical Social Work Practice*, Essential Clinical Social Work Series,
https://doi.org/10.1007/978-3-030-87783-5_2

that it may be a much older relationship, starting 40,000 years ago, but there is limited information to confirm this) (Ostrander et al., 2017).

Researchers believe that the canine–human bond began when wolves or hyenas began approaching the camps of humans to scavenge for discarded food scraps. Soon both humans and canines found the relationship could be mutually beneficial: Wolves would help the humans hunt and protect them from other predators, and humans would feed the wolves and bring them to their caves and fire to warm themselves (Frank & Frank, 1982). What began as a mutually beneficial working relationship soon transformed into a symbiotic relationship, with each species depending on the other for its own well-being. The breeding of wild canids for desirable traits, such as a good temperament, caused them to evolve into a different species, what we now know as the domestic dog (*canis familiaris*) (Frank & Frank, 1982). Interestingly, unlike the evolution of other domesticated species, the domestication of wild canids to domestic dogs appears to have happened in multiple places around the world at the same time (Ostrander et al., 2017).

The symbiotic relationship between dogs and humans continues to this day and is unique among interspecies relationships. Dogs have become extremely adept at reading human emotions and body language, and they have also become very dependent. Dogs depend on humans for their basic needs, such as food and shelter; they are also strikingly attuned to human emotions and body language. Recent research shows that dogs are able to read social cues from humans that wolves, primates, and other species are unable to understand (Hare & Tomasello, 2005). When researchers pointed at a hidden reward, dogs were able to find the reward immediately. Dogs were also able to follow the gaze of a researcher to locate the hidden reward. Wolves were more adept at using environmental cues to find the hidden objects, but were unable to understand or interpret human body language effectively enough to find the object using human direction (Hare et al., 2002). The evolution of dogs from wolves gave them this ability to understand human direction (primates, who are most closely biologically related to humans, were unable to follow human directions, suggesting it is an evolutionary trait, not a genetic one). This ability to innately tune in to the physical and psychological needs of humans is what makes dogs, as a species, especially well-suited to work as therapy, emotional support, or service animals.

The domestic cat (*felis catus*) is one of the most common pets found in households. The modern pet cat is descended from wild cats and, unlike dogs, they have retained many of their wild qualities despite domestication. Driscoll et al. (2009) suggest that the domestication of cats began in the Middle East when people started moving from the countryside to larger villages (approximately 10,000 years ago). When the people started forming more urban-style dwellings, they encountered a problem: They had to store enough food to feed the inhabitants of the city, but rodents and insects would invade the grain stores. Dogs, as omnivores and scavengers by nature, were not suited to guard the food because they, themselves, would consume the stored food. Cats, however, are obligate carnivores and showed little interest in consuming grains (Serpell, 2000). They were more interested in catching and consuming the pests that were invading the grain stores, leaving the grain safe for human consumption. This is yet another example of a mutually beneficial relationship between humans and another species of animal.

Eventually, cats moved from being a primary source of pest control to a beloved pet. In ancient Egypt, cats were revered and regarded as godlike and divine; many cats received elaborate burials when they passed away (or were buried alive with their human guardians) (Driscoll et al., 2009). However, as affectionate and loving as cats may be, they never psychologically evolved in the same way that dogs did, and they remain less able (or less interested) in understanding human social cues (Miklósi et al., 2005). It is this independent nature that endears them to many of us, since they retain their wild roots even as they provide affection and attention to their human guardians. Cats continue to be involved in pest control for many people, guarding stores of food all over the world, but their relationship with humans has developed past a working relationship to a relationship that is often primarily emotional.

Just as with dogs and cats, the relationship between horses (*equus caballus*) and humans started as a working relationship and quickly developed into an emotional attachment. When we think of large animals, it is usually not as companion animals. Domestication as it applies to large animals can be defined in several ways, either by human control over breeding the animal (for desirable traits) or by the utilization of the animal for human purposes (Russell, 2002). Whichever definition is used, scientists suspect that horses were first kept by people around 3500 BC (Goodwin, 1999). It is believed that originally horses were kept as a meat source, but then they became integral in transportation (including pulling chariots), agriculture, and warfare. Interestingly, we still today find working horses in major cities, where they are involved in police work and in pulling carriages, despite industrialization and more modern forms of transport.

Horses are the only species other than dogs that, according to the Americans with Disabilities Act, are legally acceptable to work as service animals in the United States (Clark, 2016). This is because horses, like dogs, read body language exceptionally well (sometimes for their own safely, not just ours) and are adept at reading human social cues. The story of Clever Hans is a prime example of this skill. In 1907, in Germany, a horse named Hans was thought to be so intelligent that he could solve complex math problems (Beran, 2012). His owner would ask him a math question and Hans would stamp out the answer with his foot. Hans and his owner became very famous and people were in awe of the intellectual abilities of this horse. However, eventually it was revealed that Hans could not do math at all. Hans was actually very adept at reading human body language and social cues, and would figure out the answer to the math problem by reading the body language of those around him. Humans have involuntary behaviors that they often are not consciously aware of and studies show that between 65% and 95% of human communication is nonverbal in nature (Matsumoto et al., 2012). Although fans of Clever Hans were disappointed that he could not do math, his skill at reading human body language, the nonverbal communication of another species, certainly was extraordinary. As with dogs, the relationship between humans and horses became symbiotic over time, moving from a working relationship to a more emotional bond (Beran,

2012). Today, hippotherapy (equine therapy) is an effective treatment modality that is used today to treat many conditions, from physical ailments such as neurological problems to disorders of the mind such as autism, depression, anxiety, and trauma (Koca & Ataseven, 2015).

Of course, HAB is not limited to these three species. There are reports of spontaneous relationships forming between wild animals and humans. In Brazil, a pod of dolphins has learned to work cooperatively with the local fishermen; the dolphins will herd fish into the fishing nets and, in return, the fishermen will feed the dolphins (Cantor et al., 2018). Pet Partners, a national advocacy organization, lists several additional species of animals that are appropriate for therapy work such as llamas, pigs, and rabbits (Compitus, 2021). Even if an animal is not suited for formal work as a therapy animal or service animal, a person may form an emotional bond with a pet and receive a therapeutic benefit from interacting with that pet.

Animals in Therapy

Although animal-assisted therapy is a burgeoning field only emerging into the sphere of public awareness, people have known about the therapeutic benefits of human–animal interactions for centuries. In the late 1600s, the world-famous philosopher John Locke suggested that spending time with animals aided the social development of children and was important in the development of empathy (Locke, 1887; Ritvo, 1985). Animals were integrated into some of the first prototypes of modern therapeutic models in the eighteenth century; the first documented, intentional use of animals in therapy took place in 1792, at a Quaker clinic in England (Cole & Howard, 2013). The clinic housed mentally ill patients and staff discovered that when the patients cared for the animals at the facility it aided in their recovery. In the 1870s, a Paris surgeon began having his patients with neurological conditions ride horses to improve their motor control and balance (Berg & Causey, 2014). He quickly noticed that the patients who were involved in this early form of equine therapy were less likely to suffer from depression than his other patients. Famed nineteenth-century nurse Florence Nightingale also integrated animals into her treatment plan, noting that interacting with small pets helped alleviate depressive symptoms in her patients (Hooker et al., 2002).

Possibly the most famous, and surprisingly little recognized, animal-assisted therapist was Sigmund Freud (Zilcha-Mano et al., 2011), who began integrating his Chow dogs into client sessions to relieve his own symptoms of anxiety when working with difficult cases (Ernst, 2014). Freud transcribed his observations on the benefits of animal-assisted therapy, though they were never widely published. He observed that both therapist and patients appeared more relaxed when an animal was in the room. He discovered that children and adolescents were more willing to speak openly about difficult issues when his dog was in a room (Chandler, 2017). Freud believed that animals have a "special sense" allowing them to accurately judge a person's character. He wrote specifically about his dog, Jofi, who could signal a patient's level of tension by where he lay in the room; Jofi would move closer to the patient if they were less tense and would sit farther away if the person was more tense (Ernst, 2014). As many dogs do, Jofi also was said to have an innate sense of time and would signal when a session was over by pawing at the door to go out (Siporin, 2012).

Although there is a long history of dogs assisting blind people, the first formal service dog program is less than a century old. Developed in Germany after World War I, it did not last very long (Ostermeier, 2010), but other schools eventually followed. When American Morris Frank received a guide dog named Buddy from a program in Switzerland (Fishman, 2003), he was inspired to establish the first guide dog school in the United States in 1929. He called it "The Seeing Eye" (technically, all "seeing eye dogs" should come from this particular agency, although now the term has become synonymous with any guide dog for a blind person) (Fishman, 2003). In 2010, The Seeing Eye celebrated their 15,000th pairing of a blind person with a trained guide dog (Ostermeier, 2010). Since its inception, the organization has "played an integral part in shaping public policy guaranteeing access and accommodation to people who use service animals" (The Seeing Eye, n.d.).

Despite Freud's early observations, it wasn't until the 1960s that animals' potential role in mental health services began to be more formally explored. Boris Levinson was a pediatric psychologist who, like Freud, accidentally discovered the therapeutic benefits of having an animal integrated into formal mental health treatment plans; in this case, Levinson's dog Jingles was present during sessions with a pediatric patient. Levinson wrote extensively about his work in animal-assisted therapy and he is now known as the father of clinical AAT (Ernst, 2014).

Levinson's patient was a 9-year-old boy who had become increasingly socially withdrawn. Levinson noted that when Jingles was present in the session, the boy quickly became more sociable. He hypothesized that this accelerated progress was due to the dog's role in the establishment of a safe holding environment (Winnicott, 1960), which created a deeper level of trust between the therapist and the client. In 1961, Levinson presented his work to the American Psychological Association to mixed reviews; in 1969 he published his first book on AAT, entitled *Pet-Oriented Child Psychotherapy* (Ernst, 2014). Levinson's work was seminal and influenced the forming of one of the world's largest therapy animal organizations, the Delta Society (now known as Pet Partners). Levinson continued his work in AAT for many years, publishing a number of books and scientific papers on the subject.

At around the same time, an American nurse named Elaine Smith who worked at a hospital in England noticed that her patients would respond to treatment better when the chaplain visited with his dog than when he visited alone (Butler, 2013). In 1976, she formed Therapy Dogs International (TDI), and the first animal-assisted therapist visit took place in New Jersey with five handlers and six dogs (Butler, 2013). TDI has since expanded to include Disaster Stress Relief Dogs (DSRD) that are deployed to aid in emergency crisis intervention. Animal-Assisted Crisis Response (AACR) teams were first created to help people following the Oklahoma City bombing in 1995, and have since been deployed to many major crisis sites, including lower Manhattan after the World Trade Center bombing and to several school shooting sites (the benefits of AACR will be discussed in the section on crisis intervention) (Butler, 2013).

In the months preceding this book's publication, animals have filled a new therapeutic role: During the COVID-19 pandemic, many people who were stuck at home in quarantine or following lockdown orders adopted or purchased companion animals in an attempt to alleviate their feelings of isolation, loneliness, depression, and anxiety. This included a migration of adoptable animals from the southern part of the United States up north, similar to the transportation of adoptable animals after Hurricane Katrina (Phillips, 2020). Although many new pet guardians report feeling comforted by their new family member, the adoption of animals should not be perceived as a panacea. Pet/guardian relationships should be understood in terms of guardian responsibility and mutual benefit, and not entered into hastily; there remains debate as to whether the pandemic has helped or hurt the welfare of companion animals (Parry, 2020).

Nearly 400 years after Locke noted the benefits of HAB, the field of clinical animal-assisted therapy is only beginning to come into its own. Most notably, social work schools have started offering courses on HAB or veterinary social work to their students. Despite the rise in interest in AAT, there remain few certification programs available to clinicians interested in learning more about this modality. Currently, one of the most well-established certification programs is located at the International Institute for Animal Assisted Play Therapy®, founded by Risë VanFleet and Tracie Faa-Thompson. Other notable clinicians working in the field include Aubrey Fine, James A. Serpell, Cynthia Chandler, and Leslie Irvine. There has also been increasing interest in HAB from Animal Studies scientists, most notably Temple Grandin, who has written extensively about the benefits of HAB to people with Autism Spectrum Disorder.

Several scientific journals and organizations dedicated to anthrozoology have focused on publishing and disseminating ongoing research into the benefits of HAB for people and therapy animals. These include *Anthrozoös*, an international scientific journal focused on chronicling the effects of human–animal interactions across a variety of areas such as anthropology, medicine, psychology, and zoology; and ISAZ, the International Society of Anthrozoology. Another large agency, HABRI (the Human–Animal Bond Research Institute), has developed a catalogue of HAB studies and a grant program for those interested in adding to the body of scientific research on AAT and HAB. Even the National Institutes of Health (NIH) now provides grants for research on AAT.

Most current research in the field comes from psychologists, psychiatrists, and animal scientists; social workers, as yet, are not well represented. An exception is the collaboration between the Urban Resource Institute and the ASPCA in the creation of the URI/PALS program to study the needs of domestic violence victims and their pets (this program will be discussed more in the crisis intervention chapter). Although not specific to social work, Frankie's Friends provides grants to study the way veterinary care is provided to pets. Despite the rise in veterinary social work programs, and the fact that many social workers have been integrating HAB into their work for many years, there remains a gap in the research on clinical social workers helping people with pets. Most grants, such as the NIH grants, tend to focus on direct applications of AAT and neglect the importance of recognizing that every concrete service provided has the potential for a clinical interaction. Social workers have a tradition of working with the person-in-environment, and that is why it is critical that we expand our research base to include the amazing work that social workers are already doing to help clients with pets.

References

Beran, M. (2012). Did you ever hear the one about the horse that could count? *Frontiers in Psychology, 3*, 357.

Berg, E. L., & Causey, A. (2014). The life-changing power of the horse: Equine-assisted activities and therapies in the US. *Animal Frontiers, 4*(3), 72–75.

Butler, K. (2013). *Therapy dogs today: Their gifts, our obligation*. Dogwise Publishing.

Cantor, M., Simões-Lopes, P. C., & Daura-Jorge, F. G. (2018). Spatial consequences for dolphins specialized in foraging with fishermen. *Animal Behaviour, 139*, 19–27.

Chandler, C. K. (2017). *Animal-assisted therapy in counseling*. Taylor & Francis.

Clark, J. R. (2016). A horse is a horse, of course, of course. *Air Medical Journal, 35*(2), 63–64.

Cole, M., & Howard, M. (2013). Animal-assisted therapy: Benefits and challenges. In *Biotherapy-history, principles and practice* (pp. 233–253). Springer.

Compitus, K. (2021). The process of integrating animal-assisted therapy into clinical social work practice. Clinical Social Work Journal, *49*(1), 1–9.

Degerbøl, M. (1961, December). On a find of a preboreal domestic dog (Canis familiaris L.) from Star Carr, Yorkshire, with remarks on other Mesolithic dogs. In *Proceedings of the Prehistoric Society* (Vol. 27, pp. 35–55). Cambridge University Press.

Driscoll, C. A., Clutton-Brock, J., Kitchener, A. C., & O'Brien, S. J. (2009). The taming of the cat. *Scientific American, 300*(6), 68.

Ernst, L. (2014). Animal-assisted therapy: an exploration of its history, healing benefits, and how skilled nursing facilities can set up programs. *Annals of long-term care: Clinical care and aging, 22*(10), 27–32.

Fishman, G. A. (2003). When your eyes have a wet nose: The evolution of the use of guide dogs and establishing the seeing eye. *Survey of Ophthalmology, 48*(4), 452–458.

Frank, H., & Frank, M. G. (1982). On the effects of domestication on canine social development and behavior. *Applied Animal Ethology, 8*(6), 507–525.

Goodwin, D. (1999). The importance of ethology in understanding the behaviour of the horse. *Equine Veterinary Journal, 31*(S28), 15–19.

Hare, B., Brown, M., Williamson, C., & Tomasello, M. (2002). The domestication of social cognition in dogs. *Science, 298*(5598), 1634–1636.

Hare, B., & Tomasello, M. (2005). Human-like social skills in dogs? *Trends in Cognitive Sciences, 9*(9), 439–444.

Hooker, S. D., Freeman, L. H., & Stewart, P. (2002). Pet therapy research: A historical review. *Holistic Nursing Practice, 17*(1), 17–23.

Koca, T. T., & Ataseven, H. (2015). What is hippotherapy? The indications and effectiveness of hippotherapy. *Northern Clinics of Istanbul, 2*(3), 247.

Larson, G., Karlsson, E. K., Perri, A., Webster, M. T., Ho, S. Y., Peters, J., Stahl, P. W., Piper, P. J., Lingaas, F., Fredholm, M., Comstock, K. E., Modiano, J. F., Schelling, C., Agoulnik, A. I., Leegwater, P. A., Dobney, K., Vigne, J.-D., Vilà, C., Andersson, L., & Lindblad-Toh, K. (2012). Rethinking dog domestication by integrating genetics, archeology, and biogeography. *Proceedings of the National Academy of Sciences, 109*(23), 8878–8883.

Locke, J. (1887). Some thoughts concerning education. CUP Archive.
Matsumoto, D., Frank, M. G., & Hwang, H. S. (Eds.). (2012). *Nonverbal communication: Science and applications*. Sage.
Miklósi, Á., Pongrácz, P., Lakatos, G., Topál, J., & Csányi, V. (2005). A comparative study of the use of visual communicative signals in interactions between dogs (Canis familiaris) and humans and cats (Felis catus) and humans. *Journal of Comparative Psychology, 119*(2), 179.
Ostermeier, M. (2010). History of guide dog use by veterans. *Military Medicine, 175*(8), 587–593.
Ostrander, E. A., Wayne, R. K., Freedman, A. H., & Davis, B. W. (2017). Demographic history, selection and functional diversity of the canine genome. *Nature Reviews Genetics, 18*(12), 705.
Parry, N. M. (2020). COVID-19 and pets: When pandemic meets panic. *Forensic Science International: Reports, 2*, 100090.
Phillips, M. M. (2020). Coronavirus panic buying: Puppies. *The Wall Street Journal*. Retrieved from https://www.wsj.com/articles/coronavirus-makes-us-upset-puppies-are-coming-to-the-rescue-11586530110
Ritvo, H. (1985). Learning from animals: Natural history for children in the eighteenth and nineteenth centuries. *Children's Literature, 13*(1), 72–93.
Russell, N. (2002). The wild side of animal domestication. *Society & Animals, 10*(3), 285–302.
Serpell, J. A. (2000). Domestication and history of the cat. In *The domestic cat: The biology of its behaviour* (Vol. 2, pp. 180–192). Cambridge University Press.
Siporin, S. (2012). Talking horses: Equine psychotherapy and intersubjectivity. *Psychodynamic Practice, 18*(4), 457–464.
The Seeing Eye. (n.d.). *History*. Retrieved on December 12, 2020 from https://www.seeingeye.org/about-us/history.html
Winnicott, D. W. (1960). The theory of the parent-infant relationship. *International Journal of Psycho-Analysis, 41*, 585–595.
Zilcha-Mano, S., Mikulincer, M., & Shaver, P. R. (2011). Pet in the therapy room: An attachment perspective on animal-assisted therapy. *Attachment & Human Development, 13*(6), 541–561.
Compitus, K. (2021). The process of integrating animal-assisted therapy into clinical social work practice. *Clinical Social Work Journal, 49*(1), 1-9.

Chapter 3
The Biopsychosocial Model as a Framework for Understanding the Human–Animal Bond

As a clinical social worker, I use a biopsychosocial framework to examine the basic tenets of the human–animal bond (HAB). The biopsychosocial model is an interdisciplinary model that considers the interaction of biology, psychology, and the social environment as a framework to explain human development, health, and illnesses (Griffiths, 2005). This is an appropriate model to use in understanding HAB, as there is no single factor that can explain the therapeutic benefits of the human–animal bond. Biological factors such as hormonal changes are at play when people interact with animals, as well as a myriad of physical health benefits. In addition to the biological changes that happen as a result of our interactions with animals, our mental state, feelings, cognitions, and behavior also may change. We adapt our psyche to accommodate the needs of our pets and, in turn, we adapt our psyche to our lives with them. Biology and psychology can be considered individually, but as social workers, we prioritize the idea of the person-in-environment, which takes both into account. Equally, the social environment is pivotal to the social worker's understanding of human experience. Eradicating social isolation, a life-threatening scourge, is among the Grand Challenges for Social Work initiated by the American Academy of Social Work and Social Welfare. HAB can help address this and other societal challenges, given that pets help people build communities while remaining connected to each other. Throughout the book I will be referring back to the biopsychosocial framework of HAB, because it is the most fitting lens to look through when considering the possible ways that animals enrich our lives.

Biological

There are several medical benefits to pet guardianship. The benefits of animal companionship on physiological ailments like blood pressure, coronary artery disease, and diabetes are long-established (Beetz et al., 2012; Knight & Edwards, 2008;

K. Compitus, *The Human-Animal Bond in Clinical Social Work Practice*, Essential Clinical Social Work Series,
https://doi.org/10.1007/978-3-030-87783-5_3

O'Haire, 2010). Research shows that people with pets are likely to exercise more than the average person, lowering the risk of heart disease and diabetes (Maranda & Gupta, 2016). Of course, those with pets that require long walks (such as dogs) are more likely to get these particular health benefits, rather than those with pets that mostly stay inside such as hamsters or lizards. In addition, there are further variables that will determine how much exercise a person gets, such as motivation and physical location; for example, those with dogs in rural areas may have their dogs run in a yard, while city-dwellers likely have to walk their dog at least three times a day for bathroom breaks and to ensure the animal gets adequate exercise. However, this health benefit is only one of many pet guardians may enjoy.

Meta-analyses of the health outcomes of pet owners also reveal that people with pets may recover more quickly from surgery, have lower cortisol levels when petting an animal (the purr of a cat in particular appears to be biologically soothing to humans), and may even have lower cholesterol levels, heart rates, and blood pressure, which suggests improved cardiovascular health (McNicholas et al., 2005). There is even some evidence for the reduction of stress-related chemicals in the body such as epinephrine and norepinephrine, as well as evidence of an improvement in pain management (Beetz et al., 2012).

Crucially, pets also seem to influence humans' oxytocin levels. Oxytocin is a hormone that helps people form emotional connections; it is often found in mothers and their infant children as well as in romantic partners. Oxytocin makes people feel good, and due to the influence of the hormone on emotional connections it is often referred to as the "love hormone." When people who love each other are together, be it mothers and children, significant others, or good friends, their oxytocin levels rise due to the pair-bonding effect (Zik & Roberts, 2015). Other oxytocin effects include an increase in social interaction (since people are more inclined to socially bond with others) and a decrease in aggression (Berends et al., 2019). (When people end a relationship, part of the pain they feel is the result of a chemical withdrawal from oxytocin as those levels are depleted [Field, 2017]). Interestingly, research shows that when people spend time with animals, their oxytocin levels also go up, as does the oxytocin level of the animal (Beetz et al., 2012). This would suggest that spending time with animals makes us feel good and they also similarly enjoy spending time with us. The same study also showed that when people were reunited with their own pet, their oxytocin level was higher than when they spent time with an animal unfamiliar to them. This offers evidence that people's bonding with their pets creates a similar chemical response to their bonding with specific humans.

Recent studies have looked at the use of oxytocin as a psychopharmaceutical to treat people with attachment disorders, such as borderline personality disorder (Herpertz & Bertsch, 2015), since it makes people feel more emotionally secure and generally content.

The raised levels of oxytocin in humans when interacting with their own pets thus suggests that pets may provide a reparative or replacement attachment bond, similar to the psychic holding environment described by D.W. Winnicott (1960).

Psychological

There are several psychological theories that may explain why we bond to animals so deeply. As mentioned earlier, Winnicott was influential in the development of object relations theory (Tonnesmann, 2018), which is one of the primary theoretical frameworks of the human–animal bond, along with attachment theory and self-psychology. I will start chronologically, with a discussion of attachment theory and the work of Bowlby and Ainsworth as it applies to the human–animal bond. I will then move into a discussion of object relations theory and finish this section with an explanation of HAB in self-psychology. These are by no means the only psychological theories that apply to HAB, since all human behavior can be understood in terms of Maslow's hierarchy of needs (Hopper, 2019) or Bronfenbrenner's ecological systems model (Tudge & Rosa, 2019) and the human–animal bond can certainly be examined through a psychoanalytic or Gestalt lens. However, I believe that the ecological and developmental models are best discussed in a social context, while the psychology of HAB is best understood first in terms of how people attach to animals, and this understanding can form the basis for clinicians' individual work.

"Attachment" can be defined as a deep and enduring emotional bond that connects one person to another and is not restrained by space or time (Cohen, 1974). Attachment Theory, as developed by Ainsworth and Bowlby, postulates that humans are driven to form close relationships to one another in various social forms (romantic, familiar, platonic, etc.) (Ainsworth & Bowlby, 1991; Bowlby & Ainsworth, 2013). Studies have found that the desire to form relationships with animals is very similar to the way humans develop relationships to each other (Cohen, 2002; Thielke & Udell, 2017). Attachment may be characterized by specific behaviors in children, such as seeking proximity to an attachment figure (parent, sibling, teacher, etc.) when they are upset or feel threatened (Ainsworth, 1979). This explains how the parent–child relationship develops and how this relationship, in turn, influences subsequent psychological attachments. According to Bowlby, all infants have a drive to move close and seek safety and security from an attachment figure when they are under stress or feel threatened; this person is often called the "safe base" (Bowlby, 1982). It is important to note that this attachment is not based on who provides sustenance (food) to the child, as previously believed, but that it is based on the one who plays, interacts, and communicates with the child. We now understand that the responsiveness of the attachment figure to the child may be the key to the attachment (Ainsworth et al., 1974). This relationship, as stated above, is not restricted to human children and caretakers. The relationship between a pet and their guardian is very similar to the attachment formed between humans, since the relationship is reciprocal, dynamic and based on the well-being of both the human and the pet (Field et al., 2009). Humans often report that they feel their pet is their "safe base," since pets may provide both psychological and physical safety (Compitus, 2019; Compitus, 2021). Studies show that pets may be instrumental in helping people recover from grief due to loss, since they appear to be loving and supportive in an unconditional and nonjudgmental way (Kurdek, 2008, 2009).

Attachment is an adaptive trait in people and animals, since it enhances a (human or animal) infant's chance of survival. This trait is best illustrated in Konrad Lorenz's study of imprinting (Hess, 1959) and Harry Harlow's study of attachment in infant monkeys. Harlow was one of the first to debunk the theory that attachment comes from the one who provides food to the infant. He provided infant monkeys with fake "mothers," one that was made of wire and provided food, and another that was made of soft cloth and didn't provide food (Harlow & Zimmermann, 1959). Harlow found that the baby monkeys were drawn to the cloth mothers for comfort and would only go to the wire mothers to eat. Harlow explained this phenomenon by stating that attachment develops as the result of someone providing "tactile comfort" that infants have an innate biological need to touch and hold something for emotional comfort, and that emotional attachment appears to be more important for survival than even food. In his landmark study, under duress, the baby monkeys would cling to the cloth mother and this tactile stimulation would decrease their stress levels (Harlow & Zimmermann, 1959); (which means that) it is the sensitive response and security provided by the caregiver, not the provision of food, that is of primary importance in building attachment, and attachment is a natural response, especially in times of stress. In HAB, we have noted that when humans pet or stroke an animal, the tactile stimulation may trigger a psychological reaction similar to being with a caregiver and provides a method to de-stress and regain a state of equilibrium during trying times (which is one of the theories behind animal-assisted crisis response).

Lorenz also studied the mechanisms of attachment when he considered the attachment of some species of animals to the first large moving object they met after birth; he described this term as "imprinting" (Hess, 1959). The theory of imprinting suggests that attachment is innate, genetically programmed, and required for species survival. Combining the animal and human theories of attachment to understand it as a biopsychological process, we may hypothesize that children come into the world biologically programmed to form attachments with others in order to optimize survival rates. Bowlby elaborated on this theory by suggesting that a child would initially form only one primary attachment, and that the attachment figure acted as a secure base to which the child could always return after exploring the potentially scary world. This primary attachment figure then serves as the prototype for all future social relationships (Waters et al., 2002). In humans, there are four styles of attachment: secure (autonomous), avoidant (dismissing), anxious (preoccupied), and disorganized (unresolved) (Waters et al., 2002). It is important for the AAT and HAB clinician to keep these attachment styles in mind when working with clients, since the attachment style that a human has developed in response to their primary childhood caretaker can affect how they interact with other humans as an adult. It can also influence how adults interact with animals, and it is important to note that not all attachment styles will respond to AAT in the same way. For example, those with an avoidant style may have no interest in forming a relationship with animals, while those with an anxious style may hesitate to bond with a pet because of their shortened lifespan (and fears the animal will die/abandon the person).

Those with a disorganized attachment style may actually be the most responsive to AAT interventions, since an animal companion may provide them with the secure attachment that they did not have as a child and interacting with an animal may serve as a reparative relationship. Herpertz and Bertsch (2015) examined the role of oxytocin in people diagnosed with Borderline Personality Disorder. They found that people with a disrupted parent–child attachment history could benefit from treatment with oxytocin. Since a bond with a pet has been determined to stimulate a natural oxytocin production, we can assume that the human–animal bond has a twofold effect on those with a disorganized attachment style; it provides both a psychological (safe base) reparative effect and a biological (hormonal) benefit. Jasperson (2010) also considered the therapeutic benefits of AAT in working with female inmates diagnosed with disorganized and insecure attachment styles, and found that inmates were more likely to engage in group discussions and activities when a therapy animal was present at the session (Jasperson, 2010). Participants reported feeling more engaged in therapy, feeling more socially confident, and practicing improved boundary setting as a result of engaging in animal-assisted group therapy. Of course, AAT's benefits do not apply only to those with an insecure attachment style; I am only suggesting that this particular population may especially benefit from AAT. (Comorbid disorders should also be considered when assessing a client for AAT, and this will be discussed in a future chapter.)

Object relations is another theoretical lens through which to understand the human–animal bond. Object relations is an offshoot of psychoanalytic theory, which focuses on a person being motivated by a need for connection to others (rather than by Freud's innate drives). A discussion of object relations often starts with an analysis of the family of origin (especially the mother–child dyad). The word "object" refers not to inanimate objects but to any significant other to whom the client forms an emotional connection (Fairbairn, 1963). This is usually a mother, father, or primary caregiver, but may also be a pet. An "object" may also refer to a mental representation of a primary caregiver (a "part"), and some clinicians may prefer to understand the human–animal bond as a client's mental representation of their relationship with a caregiver as transferred onto a pet. The term "relations" refers to the relationship between the client and others and the way that past relationships (especially with their primary caretaker) influence the client's current interpersonal relationships (Fairbairn, 1963). Therefore, object relations theorists study the ways that inner images of the self and the other shape interpersonal situations. HAB can easily be dissected through an object relations lens, since the relationship that a person has with their pet often mimics the relationships that they have had with other humans.

Winnicott (1960) often used the term "holding" as referring to not just a mother's physical holding of a child, but the psychological holding of emotional space for the child. When a clinician holds space for a client, they are providing the client a safe space in which to express their emotions, without judgment or conditions. Pets may provide their people with emotional holding as well, since people often perceive their pets as unconditionally loving, supportive, and nonjudgmental (Compitus, 2019; Compitus, 2021). Another term that Winnicott popularized is "the transitional object," which may refer to any "object" (person, place, pet, or thing) that mentally represents a primary love object (often the primary caretaker from childhood) (Litt, 1986). Transitional objects in childhood are commonly a beloved blanket or stuffed animal, something the child can carry with them that allows them to hold a memory of their mother (or other primary caretaker) and provides them the sense of safety and security that they feel when they are with her, as well as lessening the distress of separation (Winnicott, 1986). Pets may be viewed as a transitional object, since they may provide their person with a sense of safety, security, and unconditional love, the same emotions that should develop between a child and their caretaker. The relationship with the pet, therefore, mimics that of the child and mother, and this is why the pet may be known as a "transitional object." However, some clinicians feel that this position puts the pet in a secondary role, whereas pets may certainly be viewed as a primary love object for some clients.

Self-psychology is another theoretical lens that may be used to view HAB. Self-psychology focuses on the development of empathy in a client, the fundamental components of healthy development and growth, and a sense of self. Self-psychology postulates that in an appropriate environment a child will develop a healthy sense of self; if a healthy environment is not available, a child may grow to rely on others ("self-objects") to get their emotional needs met (Brown, 2004). "Transference" is when the client redirects (or transfers) their feelings or desires for one person to an entirely different living being, such as the therapist or a beloved pet. A client who has not received appropriate emotional support as a child may then transfer their feelings of emotional dependency onto the animal (in the way that they would feel dependent on a caregiver). Alternately, the client may project themselves onto the animal, who is physically dependent on the client to have their basic needs met (food, water, shelter, etc.) and give the animal love that they (the client) would like to have received as a child. Or, according to self-psychology, the pet may also serve as a self-object, which may be defined as a being or object that is experienced in the service of the self or as a part of and provide a particular function for the self; pets are very good at helping people with a poor sense of self regulate their emotions and self-soothe (Brown, 2004). As stated above, simply petting a purring cat lowers cortisol levels and lowers blood pressure; a purring cat, then, serves well as a self-object to help a client return to a state of equilibrium when they are decompensating.

Social Environment and HAB

In addition to biological and psychological factors, HAB must be understood in the larger context of our society. One of the most relevant facts about that larger context is that Americans are feeling increasingly alone in the world (McPherson et al., 2006). Regular and meaningful contact with other human beings—and the absence thereof—has a profound impact on physical and mental health. The impetus for social workers to address social isolation has never been clearer: Long-term impacts of social isolation are indisputable and range from minor physical illnesses and mental health issues to mortality (Shor & Roelfs, 2015). Socially isolated adults watch more TV (Van Cauwenberg et al., 2014), are more physically sedentary, and are more likely to smoke cigarettes, drink heavily, and eat un-healthfully (Schrempft et al., 2019). Older adults, due to both physical frailty and a shrinking social network, are at particular risk for both social isolation and its negative effects (Johnson & Bibbo, 2015; Peretti, 1990).

Social isolation is often conflated with loneliness, but understanding the distinction is helpful in assessment and treatment processes. As Schrempft et al. (2019) explain, social isolation is "the absence of regular contact with family and friends and lack of involvement in social organizations," while loneliness is defined as "the subjective experience or perception of being isolated." Individuals, whether due to temperament or preference, may be objectively socially isolated but not feel the subjective distress of loneliness; still, it is the nature of social isolation itself that leaves people with a mortality risk akin to smoking. While it's not firmly established why social isolation kills, it is well-established that it does, and significant research is being done to address the major causal hypotheses (House, 2001). The nature of the relationships and social connections that exist appear less important than whether they exist at all (House, 2001).

At national programmatic and policy levels within public health, we are seeing efforts to address America's growing population of socially isolated adults (McPherson et al., 2006). And yet, clinical social workers continue to witness social isolation among clients. While the reasons for it can vary—from mental illness to cognitive impairment to childcare responsibilities to incarceration (Grand Challenges for Social Work, 2015)—clinical social workers can play a unique role in helping to address this issue in their direct work with individual clients at risk for social isolation. Social isolation can be addressed by strengthening distant relationships or building additional relationships in a person's vicinity. Animal companionship ("pets") can play an important role both by improving existing human-to-human relationships and helping in the formation of new ones (Veevers, 2016). The incorporation of companion animals as a clinical intervention for social isolation is an emerging field of research, but it has been shown that companion animals can foster well-being in clients and promote opportunities to develop new social connections (Wood et al., 2015). Therefore, mental health professionals who are interested in HAB should skillfully and intentionally consider the ways that social isolation can be addressed in adults, while accounting for client attachment styles, ability to navigate the world to meet their needs, and available resources. Clinical social workers are well-trained to appropriately assess and intervene in all of these dynamics.

Historically, studies of HAB have focused primarily on the direct benefits of pet guardianship on the psychological and physiological well-being of people. McConnell et al. (2011) found that pet owners not only report higher self-esteem than the general population, but also higher levels of emotional wellness and social inclusion. However, there is a growing body of data that considers the effects of pet ownership on social communities and community health as well (Arkow, 2015), and this data shows there is often a value for the larger community when individuals have companion animals. Pets may be considered a form of "social capital" that "promotes social, economic, and physical well-being through the trusting, supportive relationships that develop" (Arkow, 2015). Messent (1983) termed the pets who facilitate social interactions between people as "social lubricants." They provide strangers with a common interest and a reason to connect and form new bonds, crucial for reducing social isolation. By establishing this common interest, pets may help people who are normally withdrawn or socially reserved to connect with others (Fine, 2017). For example, ownership of pets by community residents may encourage social conversation between neighbors. It is thus a mechanism that allows people to more quickly establish social bonds that hold larger social relationships together. These social relationships, in turn, may cause people to invest more in their community by volunteering, helping neighbors, or sharing resources, in addition to alleviating loneliness at the individual level (Wood et al., 2017).

In 2015, Wood et al. surveyed 2692 pet owners in Portland, San Diego, Nashville, and Perth, Australia to investigate how pets assisted people in growing and enhancing social networks among neighbors. Over 80% of respondents reported that, due to their pets, they had connected with neighbors that they had not previously known. Not only had they met new people, but also they formed strong social support systems that included informational support, instrumental support, appraisal support, and emotional support. Dog owners who regularly walked their pets were five times more likely to meet people through their pets, which the study's authors posited was because the pets facilitated the interaction between people. The nature of being outdoors with a pet was not the only mechanism for human-to-human connection: Owners of other types of pets (cats, fish, etc.) also reported an increase in social networking due to the shared experience of pet guardianship (Wood et al., 2015).

The establishment of trusting relationships based on animal companionship may be due to the nature of companion animals themselves. Pets are often perceived as nonjudgmental sources of support and good judges of character (author's own, in press). By extension, people who own pets are often seen in a positive light, since they appear "deserving" of the trust of the animal, thus facilitating more trusting interactions with peers. Veevers (2016) suggests that strangers may assume that pet owners are inherently friendlier people and easier to approach, thus predicting success in interpersonal human relationships.

Pet ownership may be especially helpful to older adults as their social circle narrows and/or their health declines. Pets are common companions to older adults and a strong bond may form between people and their pets (Peretti, 1990). For older adults whose adult children have moved away, pets may function as surrogate children; for those who have friends who have passed away, the pets may become surrogate friends (Veevers, 2016). Family, friends, and neighbors may be involved with the care of the pet, as well. The ownership of pets may, therefore, assist older adults in maintaining social bonds outside their homes, at a time when they may be inclined to socially withdraw. Some volunteer programs are now aimed at helping older adults care for their pets for these reasons, and many clients find it easier to accept help for their pets than for themselves (Bibbo & Proulx, 2018). The "social lubrication" or "social facilitation" effect of pets can help alleviate social isolation in older adults and people who are homebound for other reasons. Pet ownership, in summation, can be an important factor in the social functioning of older adults.

While social isolation is common in older adults (Shankar et al., 2017), it can also happen for those lacking in social skills, for the physically disabled, or for others who for various reasons find connection difficult. In such cases, pets may promote self-esteem, serve as a mechanism of communication and interaction with neighbors, and represent a healthy attachment object for the individual. However, it is contraindicated for certain individuals to become pet owners: those with severe pet allergies; those who are cognitively, physically, or financially unable to care for pets; those who live in an unsafe home environment for an animal; and those with a significant trauma history relating to animals (Compitus, 2019; Compitus, 2021).

Current trends related to the interplay of society, the environment, and HAB will be discussed in the final chapter. These include the One Health movement, broader recognition of zooeyia as a concept, and wider acceptance of pets as a social determinant of health. For now, I suggest that the numerous physiological, psychological, and social benefits emerging from HAB are becoming clearer each day as we continue to find new ways that animals create a sense of well-being in our lives.

References

Ainsworth, M. D. S., Bell, S. M., & Stayton, D. (1974). Infant-mother attachment and social development. In M. P. Richards (Ed.), *The introduction of the child into a social world* (pp. 95–135). Cambridge University Press.

Ainsworth, M. S. (1979). Infant-mother attachment. *American Psychologist, 34*(10), 932.

Ainsworth, M. S., & Bowlby, J. (1991). An ethological approach to personality development. *American psychologist, 46*(4), 333.

Arkow, P. (2015). Animal therapy on the community level: The impact of pets on social capital. In *Handbook on animal-assisted therapy* (pp. 43–51). Academic Press.

Beetz, A., Uvnäs-Moberg, K., Julius, H., & Kotrschal, K. (2012). Psychosocial and psychophysiological effects of human-animal interactions: The possible role of oxytocin. *Frontiers in Psychology, 3*, 234.

Berends, Y. R., Tulen, J. H., Wierdsma, A. I., van Pelt, J., Feldman, R., Zagoory-Sharon, O., de Rijke, Y. B., Kushner, S. A., & van Marle, H. J. (2019). Intranasal administration of oxytocin decreases task-related aggressive responses in healthy young males. *Psychoneuroendocrinology, 106*, 147–154.

Bibbo, J., & Proulx, C. M. (2018). The impact of a care recipient's pet on the instrumental caregiving experience. *Journal of Gerontological Social Work, 61*(6), 675–684.

Bowlby, J. (1982). Attachment and loss: Retrospect and prospect. *American Journal of Orthopsychiatry, 52*(4), 664.

Bowlby, J., & Ainsworth, M. (2013). The origins of attachment theory. In *Attachment theory: Social, developmental, and clinical perspectives* (Vol. 45, pp. 759–775). Routledge.

Brown, S. E. (2004). The human-animal bond and self psychology: Toward a new understanding. *Society & Animals, 12*(1), 67–86.

Cohen, L. J. (1974). The operational definition of human attachment. *Psychological Bulletin, 81*(4), 207.

Cohen, S. P. (2002). Can pets function as family members? *Western Journal of Nursing Research, 24*(6), 621–638.

Compitus, K. (2019). Traumatic pet loss and the integration of attachment-based animal assisted therapy. *Journal of Psychotherapy Integration*. https://doi.org/10.1037/int0000143

Compitus, K. (2021). The process of integrating animal-assisted therapy into clinical social work practice. *Clinical Social Work Journal, 49*, 1–9.
Fairbairn, W. R. D. (1963). Synopsis of an object-relations theory of the personality. *The International Journal of Psychoanalysis, 44*(2), 224–225.
Field, N. P., Orsini, L., Gavish, R., & Packman, W. (2009). Role of attachment in response to pet loss. *Death Studies, 33*(4), 334–355.
Field, T. (2017). Romantic breakup distress, betrayal and heartbreak: A review. *International Journal of Behavior and Research in Psychology, 5*(2), 217–225.
Grand Challenges for Social Work. (2015). http://grandchallengesforsocialwork.org/wp-content/uploads/2015/12/180604-GC-social-isolation.pdf. Retrieved April 25, 2019.
Griffiths, M. (2005). A 'components' model of addiction within a biopsychosocial framework. *Journal of Substance Use, 10*(4), 191–197.
Harlow, H. F., & Zimmermann, R. R. (1959). Affectional responses in the infant monkey. *Science, 130*(3373), 421–432.
Herpertz, S. C., & Bertsch, K. (2015). A new perspective on the pathophysiology of borderline personality disorder: A model of the role of oxytocin. *American Journal of Psychiatry, 172*(9), 840–851.
Hess, E. H. (1959). Imprinting. *Science, 130*(3368), 133–141.
Hopper, E. (2019). Maslow's hierarchy of needs explained. *Viitattu, 12*, 2019.
House, J. S. (2001). Social isolation kills, but how and why? *Psychosomatic Medicine, 63*(2), 273–274. https://doi.org/10.1097/00006842-200103000-00011
Jasperson, R. A. (2010). Animal-assisted therapy with female inmates with mental illness: A case example from a pilot program. *Journal of Offender Rehabilitation, 49*(6), 417–433.
Johnson, R., & Bibbo, J. (2015). Human–animal interaction in the aging boom. In *Handbook on animal-assisted therapy* (pp. 249–260). Academic Press.
Knight, S., & Edwards, V. (2008). In the company of wolves: The physical, social, and psychological benefits of dog ownership. *Journal of Aging and Health, 20*(4), 437–455.
Kurdek, L. A. (2008). Pet dogs as attachment figures. *Journal of Social and Personal Relationships, 25*, 247–266. https://doi.org/10.1177/0265407507087958
Kurdek, L. A. (2009). Pet dogs as attachment figures for adult owners. *Journal of Family Psychology, 23*, 439–446. https://doi.org/10.1037/a0014979
Litt, C. J. (1986). Theories of transitional object attachment: An overview. *International Journal of Behavioral Development, 9*(3), 383–399.
Maranda, L., & Gupta, O. T. (2016). Association between responsible pet ownership and glycemic control in youths with type 1 diabetes. *PLoS One, 11*(4), e0152332.
McConnell, A. R., Brown, C. M., Shoda, T. M., Stayton, L. E., & Martin, C. E. (2011). Friends with benefits: On the positive consequences of pet ownership. *Journal of Personality and Social Psychology, 101*(6), 1239.
McNicholas, J., Gilbey, A., Rennie, A., Ahmedzai, S., Dono, J. A., & Ormerod, E. (2005). Pet ownership and human health: A brief review of evidence and issues. *BMJ, 331*(7527), 1252–1254.
McPherson, M., Smith-Lovin, L., & Brashears, M. E. (2006). Social isolation in America: Changes in core discussion networks over two decades. *American Sociological Review, 71*, 353–375.
Messent, P. R. (1983). Social facilitation of contact with other people by pet dogs. In A. H. Katcher & A. M. Beck (Eds.), *New perspectives on our lives with companion animals* (pp. 37–46). University of Pennsylvania Press.
O'Haire, M. (2010). Companion animals and human health: Benefits, challenges, and the road ahead. *Journal of Veterinary Behavior: Clinical Applications and Research, 5*(5), 226–234.
Peretti, P. O. (1990). Elderly-animal friendship bonds. *Social Behavior and Personality: An International Journal, 18*(1), 151–156.
Shankar, A., McMunn, A., Demakakos, P., Hamer, M., & Steptoe, A. (2017). Social isolation and loneliness: Prospective associations with functional status in older adults. *Health Psychology, 36*(2), 179.

Shor, E., & Roelfs, D. J. (2015). Social contact frequency and all-cause mortality: A meta-analysis and meta-regression. *Social Science & Medicine, 128*, 76–86.

Thielke, L. E., & Udell, M. A. (2017). The role of oxytocin in relationships between dogs and humans and potential applications for the treatment of separation anxiety in dogs. *Biological Reviews, 92*(1), 378–388.

Tonnesmann, M. (2018). Early emotional development: Ferenczi to Winnicott. In *The elusive child* (pp. 45–57). Routledge.

Tudge, J., & Rosa, E. M. (2019). Bronfenbrenner's ecological theory. In *The encyclopedia of child and adolescent development* (pp. 1–11). Wiley.

Van Cauwenberg, J., De Donder, L., Clarys, P., De Bourdeaudhuij, I., Owen, N., Dury, S., et al. (2014). Relationships of individual, social, and physical environmental factors with older adults' television viewing time. *Journal of Aging and Physical Activity, 22*, 508–517.

Veevers, J. E. (2016). The social meanings of pets: Alternative roles for companion animals. In *Pets and the family* (pp. 11–30). Routledge.

Waters, E., Crowell, J., Elliott, M., Corcoran, D., & Treboux, D. (2002). Bowlby's secure base theory and the social/personality psychology of attachment styles: Work(s) in progress. *Attachment & Human Development, 4*(2), 230–242.

Winnicott, D. W. (1960). The theory of the parent-infant relationship. *International Journal of Psycho-Analysis, 41*, 585–595.

Wood, L., Martin, K., Christian, H., Houghton, S., Kawachi, I., Vallesi, S., & McCune, S. (2017). Social capital and pet ownership – A tale of four cities. *SSM-Population Health, 3*, 442.

Wood, L., Martin, K., Christian, H., Nathan, A., Lauritsen, C., Houghton, S., Kawachi, I., & McCune, S. (2015). The pet factor-companion animals as a conduit for getting to know people, friendship formation and social support. *PLoS One, 10*(4), e0122085.

Zik, J. B., & Roberts, D. L. (2015). The many faces of oxytocin: implications for psychiatry. *Psychiatry research, 226*(1), 31–37.

Schrempft, S., Jackowska, M., Hamer, M., & Steptoe, A. (2019). Associations between social isolation, loneliness, and objective physical activity in older men and women. *BMC public health, 19*(1), 1–10.

Fine, A. H. (2017). Standing the test of time: Reflecting on the relevance today of Levinson's pet-oriented child psychotherapy. *Clinical child psychology and psychiatry, 22*(1), 9–15.

Chapter 4
Animal-Assisted Therapy

Phase One: Preparation and Assessment

Recommended Steps in AAT Work

- Selection and Certification of Therapy Animal and Handler (Team)
- Review Animal Welfare Standards
- Review AAT Competencies
- Decide Which Therapeutic Model to Integrate (Achieve Competency)
- Intake and Assessment of the Client (Rule In/Rule Out)
- Psychoeducation with Client on AAT/AAI
- Determine Client Goals, Strengths, and Weaknesses
- Develop a Treatment Plan (including Goals and Objectives)
- Implement the Treatment Plan
- Continuously Monitor Animal Welfare
- Evaluate the Session
- Record Session Notes
- Edit Objectives/Goals as Needed

Animal-Assisted Therapy (AAT) is a highly adaptive model and, as such, can be integrated into other therapeutic modalities or used as a stand-alone model. In the introduction, I discussed the difference between AAT, Animal-Assisted Interventions (AAI), and Animal-Assisted Education (AAE) (also see List of Abbreviations in the front matter of this book). In this chapter, I will be primarily discussing AAT and, more specifically, Animal-Assisted Psychotherapy (AAP), also known as Animal-Assisted Counseling (AAC). Although AAT can be used to describe any therapeutic treatment model (such as occupational therapy) that includes an animal facilitator,

K. Compitus, *The Human-Animal Bond in Clinical Social Work Practice*,
Essential Clinical Social Work Series,
https://doi.org/10.1007/978-3-030-87783-5_4

for simplicity's sake I will continue to use the term AAT throughout this chapter to discuss the animal-assisted psychotherapeutic form.

One of the most difficult aspects of AAT is also its most appealing—the adaptive and dynamic nature of the model. There are currently no published protocols and AAT/AAC/AAP is not a manualized treatment model. This means that it is difficult for clinicians to know exactly what aspects of the treatment are most effective, which parts should be continued, and what the duration of those should be (Fine, 2019). Therefore, I suggest that clinicians consider the different orientations of AAT separately, with AAP/AAC as an adjunctive model to be used with well-established psychotherapeutic practices and other forms of AAT (crisis response, adjunctive education, occupational therapy, etc.) as integrated with each of those particular fields. However, Fine (2019) suggests that regardless of the type of therapy, there are basic tenets that should be considered when animals are integrated into any practice. He suggests that therapists should consider which benefits AAT will provide the client, above and beyond other types of clinical intervention (Fine, 2019).

Therapists should consider the variety of ways in which they can integrate the animal into the therapeutic process, and how they will adapt their regular therapeutic approach to allow for the integration of AAT (Fine, 2019). Certainly, when two types of therapy are integrated, such as DBT and AAT, the clinician will not be true to the original model itself and clinicians will not be working faithfully with the original manual. Clinicians must also be aware of the considerations of integrating an animal into the therapy process. Chandler (2017) suggests that clinicians should be conscientious about including the animals in a way that is sure to enhance the treatment process, but also to make the interaction positive for the therapy animal themselves. I will close this chapter with a consideration of therapy animal welfare issues, which certainly should be one of the first considerations for any clinician working in AAT. And before starting any AAT program, clinicians who do not own their premises should check with their landlord to ensure that animals are allowed in the building, since therapy animals do not have the same rights as service animals under the ADA.

Not all species of animals and not all pets are suited to work as therapy animals. It is important to select an animal that is suited to therapy work, based on the animal's temperament, personality, and training background. Organizations such as Pet Partners or Therapy Dogs International will evaluate an animal's potential ability to work as a therapy partner. These organizations have strict rules about the types of animals that can work in therapy and the required manners (training) the animal has, as well as how the handler works with the animal. For example, llamas, pigs, rabbits, dogs, and cats qualify as potential therapy animals but lizards do not, due to their fragile constitutions and the potential for zoonotic diseases (Pet Partners, n.d.). The breed of the animal is less important than the individual temperament of the animal (see Chap. 6 section on "Breed Specific Legislation") and the clinician should only consider an animal for therapy work if the animal enjoys interacting with people and has a calm but engaging temperament.

In this chapter, when I speak about therapy animals I am usually referring to the most common species such as dogs, cats, or rabbits. This is not with prejudice toward any particular species of animals; it is simply because the aforementioned species are most often chosen by therapists for clinical work. Any interaction with an animal can be therapeutic—I, myself, have worked with cows in direct clinical service. In this chapter, I have made a conscious decision to not discuss hippotherapy (equine/horse therapy) since PATH (Professional Association of Therapeutic Horsemanship International) and EAGALA (the Equine-Assisted Growth And Learning Association) have well-developed methods of AAT that clinicians can become trained in, if they have the means to work with larger animals. PATH was created in 1969 to promote equine-assisted service and therapeutic riding for people with special needs and is one of the largest and most well-established hippotherapy organizations worldwide (Lanning & Kreneck, 2013). EAGALA is an established therapeutic model that has been somewhat manualized and is based on the mutual cooperation, participation, and respect of all parties involved (Thomas, 2011). The aforementioned International Institute for Animal Assisted Play Therapy® also has a very strong Equine Assisted Play Therapy® program that I would recommend to any clinician interested in learning more about hippotherapy. I also do not include in this chapter some of the less reputable forms of AAT, such as dolphin-assisted therapy, that are seen by many animal scientists as harmful toward animal welfare.

Therapy animal organizations are very careful to monitor the welfare not only of future human clients and handlers, but also of the therapy animals; they require that animals are trained and managed with positive reinforcement techniques only and prong, choke, and shock collars and other aversive methods are not allowed for use with therapy animals. This is to ensure the safety of the humans *and* the therapy animals, since research shows that animals trained using pain-inducing stimuli are more likely to be reactive and potentially harm another being (Haug, 2008; Herron et al., 2009). Pet Partners' criteria for certification include: the animal must be (for most species) at least 1 year old; must have lived with the current handler for at least 6 months; must be fully vaccinated; must have no dietary restrictions; must have no history of aggression; must have good manners ("obedience skills"); must welcome interactions with strangers; and must be comfortable wearing identifying gear (Pet Partners, n.d.). This means that although all therapy animals will likely live happily as family pets, not all family pets are suited to work as therapy animals and clinicians should not assume that a beloved pet is suited to therapy work just because of their connection with the guardian, handler, or therapist.

There are no requirements per se as to how the therapy animal is obtained. I am often asked if rescue/adopted animals are suited to therapy work; in fact, it depends on whether that individual animal is suited to therapy work. Therapy animals do not have to be purchased from a breeder; there are many successful therapy animals, emotional support animals, and psychiatric service animals that were adopted from shelters. For example, my own therapy dog, Chompy Chops, was found as a stray on the South Bronx streets, starved and covered in sores, at approximately 5 years old. We picked up Chompy from the person who rescued him, fully intending to rehabilitate him and find him a home as a pet. What we found is that Chompy has an amazingly sweet temperament. He is quite goofy, good at making people laugh, and loves being around people. The fact that he was rescued from an abuse/neglect situation as an adult is, in this case, irrelevant, since his temperament is well-suited to therapy work. Other dogs I have had as puppies were simply not suited for therapy work; one is shy around strangers, another is great with women but not men. Purchasing an animal from a breeder is not a guarantee that an animal will have a temperament suited to therapy work—a responsible breeder *should* have an idea of the temperament of the parents, but this still will not guarantee that the offspring will have a similar temperament. Some of the most well-known abused dogs in current history—the pit bull terriers that were badly mistreated by football player Michael Vick—went on to become wonderful, sweet, and skilled therapy dogs (Gorant, 2011). This is due to the resilient nature of animals and their ability to live in the present. Another one of my therapy animals is a paraplegic cat. Animals with a disability or a trauma background sometimes work well as therapy animals too, since clients may develop feelings of transference toward the animal (a client once told me that "if Chompy was able to recover from being abused, maybe so can I").

Regardless of where the animal is obtained, clinicians should be prepared to invest time and money into training a therapy animal to what I like to call "basic manners." The animal must attend to the clinician's guidance, not jump on people without invitation, sit, stay, and be housebroken. The way that a clinician interacts with and works with the animal is a strong predictor of success in therapy. This is why, in addition to evaluating potential therapy animals, Pet Partners evaluates and requires training for potential handlers (often, but not always, by the clinician), emphasizing skills including an ability to read the animal's body language to recognize if they are feeling stressed, readiness to reward the animal for positive interactions, and readiness to advocate for the welfare of the therapy animal at all times (Pet Partners, n.d.). Although therapy animal certification is not required by the government or for mental health licensure, I would strongly recommend it to any practitioner who is considering working with a therapy animal since it will help ensure the safety of all involved in the treatment process.

Once the therapy animal is selected and evaluated and the handler (clinician or independent contractor) is trained in how to work with a therapy animal, the environment must be set up for therapy animal work. Therapy animal welfare will be considered in detail in the closing paragraphs of this chapter, but the animal's welfare must always be considered by the clinician. In preparation, a dog crate, bed, or other restful place should be provided for the therapy animal and the animal must have access to it at all times. This is so that the animal may escape from the client if the animal feels threatened, in distress, overwhelmed, or tired, or is accidentally injured. This is for the safety of the human clients, as well as the therapy animal, since even the sweetest animal that is hurt or in distress and unable to escape may react aggressively in order to protect themselves. Other materials that should be included in the environment are a water bowl, cleaning materials (in case of an accident), and treats or toys.

Another important part of the preparation process is evaluating and preparing a potential client for AAT work. Not all clients are suited to working with therapy animals, regardless of their clinical diagnoses, and this naturally would exclude many clients diagnosed with Antisocial Personality Disorder or those with a history of violence. Novice practitioners may want to refrain from working in AAT with clients who have a history of animal abuse, although more experienced practitioners have found high rates of success in teaching clients about depersonalization versus empathy. Nancy Parish-Plass (2013) discusses the benefits of working with clients with a history of animal abuse and at the International Institute for Animal Assisted Play Therapy® they report that animal-assisted play therapy can be highly successful when working with youths in the juvenile justice system. James Garbarino (2001) has done extensive work on counteracting youth violence and certainly when we integrate AAT, we can illustrate and model skills to help encourage empathy and decrease violence (especially when we teach youth about animal sentience). There is amazing work being done with clients with an abuse history, although I would suggest that clients who are prone to violence toward others should not be considered for traditional AAI work, but rather targeted AAT with an experienced clinician. The presence of a personality disorder is not, in itself, criterion for exclusion, since many people diagnosed with Borderline Personality Disorder have a history of self-harm with no harm to others and since those with such a disorganized attachment style often have positive outcomes when treated with AAT (Jasperson, 2013). (I have personally found that many of my clients with BPD do very well in working in AAT, since they often see the therapy animal as vulnerable as they may feel.) The decision to include or exclude an individual in AAT is, therefore, variable and left up to the clinician to determine and highly dependent on the goals and type of therapy. For example, a client with a dog phobia may not be appropriate for a psychodynamic AAT approach, but may do very well if a dog is integrated into a type of exposure therapy. Before starting AAT, potential clients should be assessed to determine if they have a fear of any specific types of animals, or any allergies that would prevent them from interacting with the therapy animal. Best practices suggest that before starting treatment with AAT, the clinician should complete a thorough assessment of each client that they are considering for the correct fit with this particular treatment model (Fine, 2019).

Although not a requirement, a clinician may want to use a validated scale during intake such as the Pet Attitude Scale (PAS) (Templer et al., 1981), which is the first published scale to measure the human–animal bond. Another option is to consider the PAS or the Short Attachment to Pets Scale (SAPS) (Marsa-Sambola, Muldoon et al., 2016), if working with pediatric or adolescent clients. The PAS contains 43 questions, each on a 7-point Likert scale that reflects both the positive and negative emotions that a person may associate with a companion animal. There are several other animal-attitude scales, each with its own unique focus, including the Animal–Human Continuity Scale (Templer et al., 2006), the Companion Animal Bonding Scale (Poresky et al., 1987), the Lexington Attachment to Pets Scale (Johnson et al., 1992), the Pet Attitude Inventory (Wilson et al., 1987), the Pet Relationship Scale (Lago et al., 1988), The Companion Animal Semantic Differential (Poresky et al., 1988), and the Miller-Rada Commitment to Pets Scale (Staats et al., 1996). The choice of instrument would depend on the nature of the use by the clinician. Many clinicians reserve these scales for research purposes and may choose to include just a few select questions to integrate into their existing intake form, as needed.

Finally, clients should be prepared for the upcoming animal-assisted therapy sessions. They should be provided psychoeducation on the process of AAT, how it is administered, and what the roles of the client, the practitioner, and the therapy animal will look like. The client's expectations of AAT should be addressed and boundaries set as to what the therapy animal may or may not do during a session. It is important that the clinician be well informed about the process of AAT in order to best inform their clients. AAT is not a miracle cure, nor is it usually used as a stand-alone modality, and the options and likely outcomes of AAT should be discussed with the client. The clinician does not have to explain every aspect of the integrative model, but should provide enough information for the client to provide informed consent for treatment. Clinicians who are unfamiliar with implementing AAT should consider seeking out additional education in this model; continuing education courses in AAT are becoming more available as interest in it grows. The National Association of Social Workers (NASW) occasionally provides training in AAT, as does PESI.com, and there are a growing number of books that may help clinicians learn. Although there are few certification programs in AAT, I can highly recommend the International Association of Play Therapy's AAPT certification program in Animal-Assisted Play Therapy (VanFleet, 2020). Of course, this certification program is for those interested in play therapy only. Other than the few certification programs, some clinicians may find the lack of a manualized format frustrating, since they are left to find their own ways to integrate AAT into more well-known treatment models.

Ways to Integrate AAT

- May be directive or nondirective
- As a behavioral reward
- In bibliotherapy
- The use of metaphors
- Skill-based (social skills, etc.)
- Modeling
- Social lubricant
- Biophilia (connecting with nature)
- In play therapy
- As therapeutic touch
- In storytelling
- To achieve developmental tasks
- To teach empathy
- As a spontaneous point of discussion

Phase Two: The Development and Implementation of an AAT-Based Treatment Plan

The flexible nature of AAT is also a strength; it means that it is highly adaptable and easily integrated with most treatment models. Some of the more common integrations are with Psychodynamic Psychotherapy, Cognitive Behavioral Therapy (CBT), and Play Therapy. Although there are different ways in which AAT can be integrated into clinical practice, the therapeutic benefits of AAT are similar across the board.

Research shows that the therapeutic alliance is the number one most salient indicator of success in therapy (Arnow et al., 2013). Animal-assisted therapy facilitates the building of a rapport with a client, which accelerates the engagement process and allows the building of a therapeutic alliance to move more quickly. Levinson (1965) suggested that an animal present during therapy may help clients overcome any anxiety they have about therapy. The client may make more generous judgments about the therapist based on their care of the animal that will help accelerate the rate of rapport building. For example, if the client sees that the therapy animal is well-cared for, they may infer that the therapist will also take good care of them.

Another benefit of having a therapy animal in the room can promote the expression of emotions that the client may otherwise hesitate to express in front of another human, for fear of stigmatization or judgment. Fine (2019) explains that animals are not just a catalyst for negative emotions but "simply having an animal in a therapeutic setting can lighten the mood and lead to smiles and laughter" (p. 211). Other than their unconditional positive regard, a therapy animal may facilitate a client's expression of emotion by interacting with clients in ways that the therapist cannot, such as when the client pets or holds the animal. This tactile interaction may stimulate the senses (in a way similar to the self-soothing techniques taught in DBT), and this may bring about a sense of safety, security, and calm in a client. Therapy animals may encourage a variety of emotions in clients, from laughter to crying, which may encourage motivational change in a client (Fine, 2019). In this way, the therapy animal may be viewed as a co-facilitator working with the therapist, rather than a tool that the therapist is using.

Research suggests that the presence of a therapy animal may work as a catalyst for discussion, and help clients feel more comfortable divulging uncomfortable information, such as a history of abuse, to the therapist. I worked with an adolescent boy who was hesitant to tell me, an adult woman, that he was sexually assaulted, even though he knew that his mother had already told me the story. When the boy hesitated to discuss the abuse with me, I encouraged him to tell Chompy, my therapy dog. The client whispered his story in my dog's ear and then felt comfortable enough to repeat it out loud to me. Another time the same client hesitated before telling me about another traumatic event, and Chompy moved to sit in front of him and looked at him with such interest (as if HE were the therapist, not me), that the boy began to laugh and, as a result, felt comfortable enough to continue telling the story.

Finally, therapy animals often assist clients in modeling desirable skills and behavior (Fine, 2019). For example, when explaining DBT skills such as mindfulness or radical acceptance, I often point out that my therapy dog does not dwell on past events nor does he worry about the future. He simply lives in the moment: When he has a toy, he enjoys his toy; when he has his dinner, he enjoys his food. Fine explains that this extends to boundary-setting; I suggest that it also extends to assertiveness skill training and social skill training, giving a client a safe way to practice such skills. Any discussion of behavior management can lead into a psychodynamic analysis of the way the client was parented, and when the client works with a therapy animal this can lead to the reenactment of a childhood stressor, but this time with the possibility of a more positive outcome.

Sample AAT Intervention with ADHD Adolescent Client (Adapted from Bruneau & Johnson, 2016)

1. Behavioral Goal: Increased focus from average to 2 min
   (a) Objective 1: Increase frustration tolerance
   (b) Objective 2: Increase goal-setting
   (c) Objective 3: Increase self-efficacy
2. Intervention: Teach the therapy animal a new skill
   (a) Select a new skill with the client
   (b) Break down the skill into smaller steps
   (c) Discuss motivation of the therapy animal (behavioral rewards)
3. Record Outcomes
4. Evaluate
5. Amend intervention for the next session (i.e., move from step one to step two)

Integration of AAT with Existing Models

Very often I am asked how exactly a clinician can integrate AAT into an existing therapy practice, since there is no manual or set description of treatment options. In 2008, O'Callaghan did an extensive study of the ways that clinicians were using AAT in their therapeutic process. Although a number of techniques were described by the 31 mental health professionals involved in the survey, there were seven techniques that were most commonly incorporated and 11 therapeutic intentions (objectives). I cannot describe every therapeutic technique or intervention in detail (that would be another book), but I will briefly describe the most commonly used techniques and intentions and then some possible ways to incorporate these into other theoretical orientations, such as CBT, Psychoanalysis, and Play Therapy.

The AAT techniques most commonly used by mental health professionals were (1) the therapist reflects on the client's relationship with the therapy animal; (2) the therapist encourages the client to interact with the therapy animal (in a tactile or verbal manner); (3) the therapist discusses the therapy animal's history with the client. These three techniques may create a reparative experience for the client, by creating a positive and supportive relationship that the client may require in their time of need (similar to a child being comforted by a parent). For example, I would often remark on how my clients were responding to my therapy dog. I would say things like, "You have lowered your voice since he came closer to you," or, "You are very gentle when you pet him." This helps the client not only become more aware of their own behavior and how others respond to changes in their behavior, but helps the client become more aware of their own body. This can lead to a deeper discussion of mindfulness, intention, or somatic healing.

The spontaneous interactions that occur between the client and the animal may be pointed out by the clinician and used to further facilitate therapeutic discussion. I had a client who once noted the therapy dog would come closer to her when she was more emotionally regulated, spoke quietly, and acted calmly, and the dog would move away when she became louder, more agitated, and decompensated. She noted that this was similar to the way that human friends and family would react to her mood swings. The dog, therefore, facilitated an awareness of her own behavior and how it affected others, which was also a motivating reason to alter maladaptive behavior patterns. It is the therapist's job, then, to bring these relational interactions to the conscious awareness of the client. When the client then moves to interact with the therapy animal, this may serve as a safe and healthy catalyst for tactile responses that may not be appropriate between a client and the therapist. For example, a client may gently hug or pet a therapy animal to comfort themselves. This will teach them not only to self-soothe, but to do so in a way that is not reliant on other humans and at a time when it may not be appropriate to hug the clinician. The third technique, explaining the therapy animal's history, may help to normalize a client's experiences and help them become hopeful about recovery. For example, a clinician may want to share with their client the history of a therapy animal who was rescued from an abusive home. A client with their own trauma history may view the therapy animal's survival and safe life as a hopeful sign that they, too, may recover from past traumas. Sharing the animal's history has the added benefit of showing the client that the therapist is creating a safe holding space (Winnicott, 1960), and may be viewed by the client as evidence that the therapist is trustworthy, since the animal is safe, secure, and happy in the care of the therapist. At other times, the therapist may incorporate animal stories/metaphors to illustrate meaning the client may make from the animal's presence (see chapter on grief counseling). In other cases, there is no direct intervention but the mere presence of the therapy animal in itself is therapeutic and a reparative relationship.

I have already mentioned some of the most common therapeutic intentions (goals/objectives) that O'Callaghan reported (2008). These were: building a rapport (the therapeutic alliance), enhancing trust, facilitating insight, modeling specific behaviors, encouraging clients to share their feelings, enhancing social skills, and facilitating feelings of safety. The presence of the therapy animal may also, in itself, be a behavioral reward and encourage the client to come back each week. I have found that adolescents are often hesitant to attend therapy (due to a fear of being stigmatized by peers), but I have heard on more than one occasion that they will return to spend time with my therapy dog. Of course, once the clients are in the room they do good work and lend themselves to the process. But the therapy animals themselves serve as a safe "excuse" and behavioral reward, especially for those who do not have the time or the means to have pets at home.

Case Example: Trauma-Informed Psychodynamic AAT with Adolescent
(Demographic information has been altered to protect the identity of the client)

Steven was a 15-year-old Puerto Rican male who was brought to therapy by his mother, following her discovery that he had been inappropriately touched by a cousin several years prior. He had been sleeping a lot, was very irritable, tearful, sad, and mostly stayed in his room playing video games. Steven's mother told me that she had been divorced from Steven's father for many years and that his father was addicted to heroin and had spent most of Steven's childhood incarcerated. Steven did not want to attend therapy, since he felt that he was "fine" and didn't need help. After the initial intake session, Steven agreed to participate in AAT, since he was not allowed to have a dog at home and he was looking forward to meeting the therapy dog, Chompy. During sessions, Steven found that interacting with a therapy dog was a great incentive to come to therapy. He enjoyed the time that he spent with Chompy and reported that he felt safe with him nearby. I discussed with Steven when he felt safe and when he didn't; Steven reported that he rarely felt safe away from Chompy. He reported that he had strong memories of his father leaving him with strangers in a dirty crack-house while he went to buy drugs. He reported that his mother was loving and kind, but often had angry outbursts. We discussed what it was like to feel safe and what safety means. We discussed ways that he could carry the feeling of safety with him, even when he was away from Chompy. Steven hesitated in therapy to tell me about the sexual abuse that he suffered. I suggested that he tell Chompy what happened, since he always felt safe with Chompy. Steven called him to his side and whispered in the dog's ear. He asked if I heard it, and I honestly said that I did not. Steven offered to tell Chompy again, but a little louder. He then told the entire story of his sexual abuse and the rejection that he felt by family members (except his mother) when he disclosed the abuse. He looked at Chompy the entire time he told his story. When he finished, he put one hand on Chompy's back and then lifted his head and looked at me. He said that he had never said that story out loud and it was a relief to get it off his chest. We then discussed the abuse, how he felt about it and how it felt to be treated like the "bad guy" by family members when he disclosed the abuse. We discussed potential action to take against his abuser (his cousin), including calling the police. He decided that he would feel most comfortable calling Child Protective Services and the police with me, his mother and Chompy in the room, so we did that. Over the next few months, we continued a psychodynamic AAT approach, discussing the past events, his unconscious interpretation of those events, and how they manifested in his current behavior. Steven eventually announced that he was feeling much better and wanted to get back to a "normal teenage life," so he paused therapy sessions. He last reported a significant decrease in depressive symptoms, had joined a sports team, and was enjoying time with his friends and a new girlfriend.

Animal Assisted Play Therapy® may involve animals of many species, from bunnies to horses, but its defining characteristic is that it incorporates play as a treatment, not just for children and families, but for people of all ages, including adults and older adults (VanFleet & Faa-Thompson, 2010, 2014, 2015, 2017). AAPT builds on many theories and the therapeutic powers of play. Occasionally, it involves the reenactment of childhood experiences (play) in a therapeutic way, but it is not restricted to that. Much of the play is symbolic and involves other developmental and psychosocial aspects, such as the expression of feelings and wishes, working on relationships, or communication skills. Research suggests that play is as integral to human happiness and well-being as shelter and emotional support (Schaefer & Drewes, 2009). In fact, play, in all species, helps us explore our world in a way that optimizes our chances of survival. Animal Assisted Play Therapy® builds on the theories of traditional play and filial therapy but also integrates a therapy animal to help increase the client's sense of safety and to enhance the therapeutic alliance (Fine, 2019). AAPT may be directive or nondirective but is often intention-based, focusing on increasing emotional awareness, self-regulation, desensitization, and problem-solving (VanFleet & Faa-Thompson, 2017). Interactive play, including games and other activities, are used to accomplish these therapeutic goals. AAPT also involves the processing and debriefing of experiences, relying less on the therapist's verbal interpretation of events and more on the experiential and relational nature of AAT and play therapy (VanFleet & Faa-Thompson, 2017).

Cognitive Behavioral Therapy, when combined with AAT, addresses some of the client's behaviors and allows the clinician to elicit thought responses (explanations of the behavior) from the client. The clinician may then use directed interactions involving the animal (e.g., brush the dog or teach the dog how to do this trick) to challenge the client's distorted cognitions and maladaptive behavior patterns (Chandler, 2017). Teaching the client to train the animal can be a therapeutic process in itself, and may provide the client with both a sense of control and mastery. Just as in manualized CBT, this should allow the client to gain insight into their behavior, motivations, and dysfunctional thought patterns, and allow the client to successfully modify their behavior and view an improved outcome. In this sense, CBT (or ERP, DBT or any behavioral model) is primarily skill-based, teaching prosocial behaviors and correcting maladaptive patterns of behavior, with the therapist working to illustrate how these behaviors are harmful and facilitating change. When a therapy animal is involved in CBT, they are involved primarily as a catalyst of change—as a behavioral motivation to change, and also as the method by which the skills are taught. For example, when the client I previously mentioned noted that the therapy dog moved away when she was agitated, I was able to use this observation to prompt a discussion and skill-based lesson on social skills training. Behavioral therapy in AAT often involves having the client teach behavioral skills to the therapy animal, and then reflecting on how their own behavior is altered in the process.

Case Example: AAT with Exposure and Response Prevention Therapy (ERP)

(Demographic information has been altered to protect the identity of the client)

Mary was a 35-year-old new mother of a 6-month-old child who worked in advertising. She lived in a house with her husband, child and their two cats. Mary had worked from home since the birth of her child, and had recently developed a strong case of contamination OCD. Mary had not touched either of her beloved cats for over a year because she was afraid that they may have eaten a mouse and would transmit a disease to her and her son. Mary was not afraid for herself as much, but as the primary caretaker of her son she was afraid that his immature immune system would not be able to fight off any illnesses. Mary did not let anyone touch her son and would not even leave her husband alone with him. She loved her husband and her cats, but was afraid that they were not "clean enough" to touch her son. Utilizing Exposure and Response Prevention (ERP), which is a type of Cognitive Behavioral Therapy (CBT), we developed a hierarchy that allowed Mary to deal with her anxiety and fear of the unknown future. We began by providing psychoeducation for Mary about ERP, CBT and AAT. We determined that her compulsions most often involved extensive hand-washing and washing of her son's clothing and bedding. We developed a treatment plan that involved response prevention (stopping the compulsions) and exposure to her trigger, which was most often the fear that animals were contaminated. We started by working with Mary in the clinic, having her interact with the therapy cat, Lilou, and not wash her hands immediately afterward. We build up the amount of time she would spend interacting with Lilou the cat and the amount of time that would pass before she would wash her hands again. When Mary habituated to working with Lilou, we had her bring her son's blanket into the clinic. Mary was instructed to place Lilou on the blanket and then bring the blanket back to her son, to lay on. Mary was also provided homework–she was told to start by sitting on the sofa where her cats often lay (something she had not done in many months) and not wash her hands or the blanket afterward. When she habituated to that she was instructed to pet one of her cats and then pick up her son. Finally, she was instructed to place her son on the cats' favorite blanket and allow the cats to interact with her son. Mary struggled with her fears and anxiety but was determined to get better and worked hard at the treatment. After a few months, Mary reported that she was able to have her son interact with the cats without feeling extreme distress. She stated that she was able to hold and pet her cats again and she was so relieved to have them back in her life. She reported that, as a result of her ERP/AAT work, she was able to allow her husband to take over some of the caretaking of her son. She also finally introduced her son to his grandparents, without fear that he would contract an illness. At our last session she stated that she recognized that playing outside was healthy for her son and she had recently taken him on a walk to the park to look at the squirrels and birds.

Psychoanalysis is one of the oldest psychotherapy models that is still in use. According to psychoanalytic theory, people are controlled by unconscious biological drives and are mostly unaware of the reasons why they behave in a certain way (Gill, 1984). Transference and countertransference are major tools in psychoanalysis, and as previously discussed, a client may see themselves in the therapy animal; in this conceptualization the therapist, as the caretaker of that animal, takes on a role similar to the client's own parent or childhood caretaker. In psychoanalytic psychotherapy assisted by animals, the client is asked to explore their subconscious motivations, anxieties, and drives based on their behavioral reactions to the therapy animal. For example, a client once told me that my therapy dog didn't like her because my dog sat closer to me and farther from her. I used this spontaneous expression of feeling to explore why the client believed that the dog didn't like her, how she felt about it, and when she had felt similarly in the past. We then involved my dog as a catalyst for discussion about anxiety and when the client had developed her social phobia (she even noted that her thought about the dog not liking her sounded like her father). In psychoanalytic AAT, the therapist's job is to help the client explore these anxious feelings and undesirable drives as they spontaneously develop in relation to the therapy animal.

As a flexible treatment model, AAT allows clinicians to get creative with how they integrate a therapy animal into their preferred modality. For example, Chandler (2017) developed an entirely different model of AAT integration that she called HART (Human–Animal Relational Model). In the HART model, the therapy animal functions as a nurturer and aid to emotional dysregulation. In HART, the therapist is the facilitator (instead of the animal) and is interpreting and observing significant relational moments between the client and the therapy animal (Chandler, 2017). One of the difficulties with AAT is that it is difficult to measure the process; we go by outcomes, which are not always indicative of internal change. Chandler's method allows therapists to evaluate its efficacy. For these reasons I find that AAPT and HART are the models that come closest to manualization. However, HART is made to blend with other relational models and AAPT combines AAT with play therapy models, so they have the benefit of continuing to be dynamic and wholly integrative.

Therapeutic Models Frequently Integrated with AAT

- Psychodynamic
- Behavioral
- Cognitive–Behavioral Therapy (CBT)
- Psychoanalysis
- Client-Centered
- Play Therapy (AAPT)
- Family Systems
- Solution-Focused
- Gestalt
- Existential
- Adlerian
- Feminist Therapy
- HART/Relational

Special Considerations: Animal Welfare Issues

Regardless of what integrative treatment model you use, one of the primary concerns of AAT should always be the welfare of the therapy animal, and the therapist should *always* think of the well-being of the therapy animal and the client simultaneously. As stated earlier, one of the reasons that therapy animal welfare is so important (besides the obvious) is that the client will see how the clinician treats the therapy animal, will interpret that behavior, and will likely base their opinion of the therapist on the way the animal is treated (as a vulnerable being, dependent on the therapist, a client may associate himself or herself with the therapy animal).

There certainly are gaps in the literature when it comes to therapy animal welfare and I encourage clinicians to become more involved in researching the effect of AAT on therapy animals. In general, most clinicians that are involved in AAT follow the animal welfare standards as delineated by the UK Government's Farm Animal Welfare Committee (FAWC) (Farm Animal Welfare Committee, 2009). The five freedoms outline the most basic animal welfare rights that all animals in captivity should have, from companion animals to animals kept in zoos. These rights include freedom from hunger and thirst; freedom from discomfort; freedom from pain, injury, or disease; freedom to express normal behavior; and freedom from fear and distress (Barber & Mellen, 2013; McCausland, 2014).

As these guidelines suggest, a therapy animal should never be forced to interact with a client or participate in a session, much less be forcefully held (even as a "hug"). A therapy animal may be encouraged to participate in a therapy session, but if they simply don't want to, they should be allowed to "opt out." Therapy animals should be provided regular meals and should have water available in the therapy office (or water breaks throughout the day). Training a therapy animal should never involve painful stimuli or aversive training methods, since animals must be allowed the freedom from discomfort. Again, there are multiple reasons to promote positive reinforcement training (or "force free training") when working with a therapy animal, foremost to ensure the safety of everyone involved, since animals that are trained using aversive, painful, or "alpha dog" methods often react with aggression toward humans (AVSAB, 2007, 2008; Todd, 2018). When a client perceives that a therapy animal is trained using harsh, punitive, or painful techniques such as shock, prong, or choke collars, the therapeutic alliance is at risk of permanent rupture; due to feelings of transference a client may see a punitive therapist who harms the animal as likely to also cause the client harm, and the trust between the client and therapist will be immediately lost. Conversely, when force-free techniques are used the therapist and therapy animal develop a mutually respectful, trusting working relationship and this will contribute to the client's building of trust with the therapist. This is why I suggest only using positive reinforcement techniques when training and working with any animal, but it is absolutely a requirement when working with any animal in a therapeutic setting.

Although building a positive and respectful relationship with the therapy animal may mostly involve mutually respectful training techniques, the freedom from pain, injury, or disease also indicates that the animal should always be vaccinated, that its health should be prioritized, and that sick or injured therapy animals should not be forced to work (again, these restrictions protect the human participants as much as the animal). The freedom to express normal behavior sounds very basic, but is of vital importance; in essence, clinicians should allow their therapy animals to act in a species-appropriate way. A dog should be allowed to act like a dog, a cat like a cat, a horse like a horse, etc. Although it sounds very obvious to some, it is surprising how often we, as humans, impose our own human behavioral expectations on other species of animals. For example, I make sure to take Chompy out for potty breaks several times per day (freedom from discomfort/to express normal behavior), I provide him with water and toys in the therapy room, and I never force him to participate in therapy sessions. We must remember that therapy animals are living beings; they are our partners and co-facilitators and they are not tools to be used by us. However, this also means that, as clinicians, we must be flexible with our treatment plans. In my experience, sometimes the most effective AAT sessions are the ones where the unpredictable happened. I once was working with a client who was discussing a serious trauma when Chompy lay down, crawled on his belly and made funny happy grunting sounds. Although this could have been disruptive, it actually provided a moment of levity in the session and allowed the client to continue speaking without feeling overwhelmed. Following the five freedoms of animal welfare allow animals to be themselves and keep them content, provisions that are essential to a successful animal-assisted therapy practice.

Finally, I would like to suggest to all clinicians who are considering integrating AAT into their practice that they first take the time to review the AAT Competencies as developed by the American Counseling Association (Stewart et al., 2016). These competencies include learning ethology and animal behavior, understanding how to train or select a therapy animal, and understanding how to adapt the therapy model to the welfare and needs of the animal (Fine, 2019; VanFleet & Faa-Thompson, 2017). The list of competencies as released by the ACA is based on extensive research into AAT and was created to ensure the safety and well-being of the client, therapist, and therapy animal. It is a summary of the standards of best practices in AAT and should be required reading for any clinician interested in working in this field.

References

American Veterinary Society of Animal Behavior (AVSAB). (2007). *AVSAB position statement: The use of punishment for behavior modification in animals*. Retrieved from http://www.avsabonline.org/avsabonline/images/stories/Position_Statements/Combined_Punishment_Statements.pdf

American Veterinary Society of Animal Behavior (AVASB). (2008). *Position statement on the use of dominance theory in behavior modification of animals*. Retrieved from https://avsab.org/wp-content/uploads/2018/03/Dominance_Position_Statement_download-10-3-14.pdf

Arnow, B. A., Steidtmann, D., Blasey, C., Manber, R., Constantino, M. J., Klein, D. N., Markowitz, J. C., Rothbaum, B. O., Thase, M. E., Fisher, A. J., & Kocsis, J. H. (2013). The relationship between the therapeutic alliance and treatment outcome in two distinct psychotherapies for chronic depression. *Journal of Consulting and Clinical Psychology, 81*(4), 627.

Barber, J. C., & Mellen, J. D. (2013). Animal ethics and welfare. In *Zookeeping: An introduction to the science and technology* (pp. 53–61). University of Chicago Press.

Bruneau, L., & Johnson, A. (2016). Fido and Freud meet: Integrating animal-assisted interventions with counseling theory. *Ideas and Research You Can Use: VISTAS 2016*. VISTAS Online

Chandler, C. K. (2017). *Animal assisted therapy in counseling* (3rd ed.). Routledge.

Farm Animal Welfare Committee. (2009). *Five freedoms*. The National Archives. Retrieved on September 1, 2020 from https://webarchive.nationalarchives.gov.uk/20121010012427/; http://www.fawc.org.uk/freedoms.htm

Fine, A. H. (Ed.). (2019). *Handbook on animal-assisted therapy: Foundations and guidelines for animal-assisted interventions*. Academic press.

Garbarino, J. (2001). Lost boys: Why our sons turn violent and how we can save them. *Smith College Studies in Social Work, 71*(2), 167–181.

Gill, M. M. (1984). Psychoanalysis and psychotherapy: A revision. *International Review of Psycho-Analysis, 11*, 161–179.

Gorant, J. (2011). *The lost dogs: Michael Vick's dogs and their tale of rescue and redemption*. Penguin.

Haug, L. I. (2008). Canine aggression toward unfamiliar people and dogs. *Veterinary Clinics of North America: Small Animal Practice, 38*(5), 1023–1041.

Herron, M. E., Shofer, F. S., & Reisner, I. R. (2009). Survey of the use and outcome of confrontational and non-confrontational training methods in client-owned dogs showing undesired behaviors. *Applied Animal Behaviour Science, 117*(1–2), 47–54.

Jasperson, R. A. (2013). An animal-assisted therapy intervention with female inmates. *Anthrozoös, 26*(1), 135–145.

Johnson, T. P., Garrity, T. F., & Stallones, L. (1992). Psychometric evaluation of the Lexington attachment to pets scale (LAPS). *Anthrozoös, 5*(3), 160–175.

Lago, D., Kafer, R., Delaney, M., & Connell, C. (1988). Assessment of favorable attitudes toward pets: Development and preliminary validation of self-report pet relationship scales. *Anthrozoös, 1*(4), 240–254.

Lanning, B. A., & Krenek, N. (2013). Examining effects of equine-assisted activities to help combat veterans improve quality of life. *Journal of Rehabilitation Research & Development, 50*(8), vii–vii.

Levinson, B. M. (1965). Pet psychotherapy: Use of household pets in the treatment of behavior disorder in childhood. *Psychological Reports, 17*(3), 695–698.

Marsa-Sambola, F., Muldoon, J., Williams, J., Lawrence, A., Connor, M., & Currie, C. (2016). The short attachment to pets scale (SAPS) for children and young people: Development, psychometric qualities and demographic and health associations. *Child Indicators Research, 9*(1), 111–131.

McCausland, C. (2014). The five freedoms of animal welfare are rights. *Journal of Agricultural and Environmental Ethics, 27*(4), 649–662.

O'Callaghan, D. (2008). *Exploratory study of animal-assisted therapy interventions used by mental health professionals*. Unpublished doctoral dissertation. University of North Texas.

Parish-Plass, N. (Ed.). (2013). *Animal-assisted psychotherapy: Theory, issues, and practice*. Purdue University Press.

Pet Partners. (n.d.). *Program requirements*. Retrieved on September 1, 2020 from https://petpartners.org/volunteer/become-a-handler/program-requirements/

Poresky, R. H., Hendrix, C., Mosier, J. E., & Samuelson, M. L. (1987). The companion animal bonding scale: Internal reliability and construct validity. *Psychological Reports, 60*(3), 743–746.

Poresky, R. H., Hendrix, C., Mosier, J. E., & Samuelson, M. L. (1988). The companion animal semantic differential: Long and short form reliability and validity. *Educational and Psychological Measurement, 48*(1), 255–260.

Schaefer, C. E., & Drewes, A. A. (2009). The therapeutic powers of play and play therapy. In *Blending play therapy with cognitive behavioral therapy: Evidence-based and other effective treatments and techniques* (pp. 3–15). Wiley.

Staats, S., Miller, D., Carnot, M. J., Rada, K., & Turnes, J. (1996). The Miller-Rada commitment to pets scale. *Anthrozoös, 9*(2–3), 88–94.

Stewart, L. A., Chang, C. Y., Parker, L. K., & Grubbs, N. (2016). *Animal-assisted therapy in counseling competencies*. American Counseling Association, Animal-Assisted Therapy in Mental Health Interest Network.

Templer, D. I., Connelly, H. J., Bassman, L., & Hart, J. (2006). Construction and validation of an animal-human continuity scale. *Social Behavior and Personality: An International Journal, 34*(7), 769–776.

Templer, D. I., Salter, C. A., Dickey, S., Baldwin, R., & Veleber, D. M. (1981). The construction of a pet attitude scale. *The Psychological Record, 31*(3), 343–348.

Thomas, L. (2011). The EAGALA model of equine assisted psychotherapy and learning. *Scientific and Educational Journal of Therapeutic Riding*.

Todd, Z. (2018). Barriers to the adoption of humane dog training methods. *Journal of Veterinary Behavior, 25*, 28–34.

VanFleet, R. (2020). *Certification in animal assisted play therapy*. The International Institute of Animal Assisted Play Therapy. Retrieved on September 1, 2020 from www.iiaapt.org

VanFleet, R., & Faa-Thompson, T. (2010). The case for using animal assisted play therapy. *British Journal of Play Therapy, 6*, 4–18.

VanFleet, R., & Faa-Thompson, T. (2014). Including animals in play therapy with young children and families. In M. R. Jalongo (Ed.), *Teaching compassion: Humane education in early childhood*. Springer.

VanFleet, R., & Faa-Thompson, T. (2015). Animal-assisted play therapy. In D. A. Crenshaw & A. L. Stewart (Eds.), *Play therapy: A comprehensive guide to theory and practice*. Guilford.

VanFleet, R., & Faa-Thompson. (2017). *Animal assisted play therapy*. Professional Resource Press.

Wilson, C. C., Netting, F. E., & New, J. C. (1987). The pet attitude inventory. *Anthrozoös, 1*(2), 76–84.

Winnicott, D. W. (1960). The theory of the parent-infant relationship. *International Journal of Psycho-Analysis, 41*, 585–595.

Chapter 5
Veterinary Social Work

Social workers may be involved in a variety of aspects of the veterinary professions. Clinicians may teach communication classes to veterinarians, since active listening and empathic responses are valuable skills to have in any service-oriented practice. Clinicians may also be involved in supportive therapy with clients in an animal hospital or clinic. There are many types of counseling that can benefit humans who have unwell pets. These include palliative care counseling, helping to make medical decisions (including euthanasia), and general support to clients who are overwhelmed and feeling stressed caring for sick pets. Other veterinary social work services include community outreach, educational services for clients, running a nonprofit that funds emergency veterinary bills for low-income pet owners, or helping people with pets secure other concrete services (such as food stamps for pet food).

Another role that social workers may fill is that of counseling the veterinary staff themselves. Veterinary professions can be extremely emotionally, physically, and financially stressful. Many people who work as vets, vet techs, or even animal rescuers may find that the constant exposure to a traumatic environment can be exhausting. Although there are multiple roles that social workers may fill in animal hospitals, this chapter focuses mostly on clinical social work addressing two sides of the same coin: the pet guardian's needs, and the needs of veterinary professionals. The first part of the chapter discusses grief counseling for pet loss, while the second part of the chapter discusses the high rate of suicides in veterinarians. Although many of these concepts also apply to animal rescuers and other animal caretakers, such as shelter workers and zookeepers, I have chosen to discuss primarily the experiences of pet guardians and veterinarians.

K. Compitus, *The Human-Animal Bond in Clinical Social Work Practice*, Essential Clinical Social Work Series,
https://doi.org/10.1007/978-3-030-87783-5_5

Grief Counseling for Pet Loss

As stated earlier, the attachment between people and their pets can be very important and often people may view their pets as a family member, a buddy, or even a surrogate child (Cohen, 2002; Raup, 1999). Clinicians may view this relationship as individual and authentic, or they may see the pet as a transitional object for the client (Compitus, 2019; Winnicott, 1969). Kurdek (2008) found that many college students reported their attachment to their pets resembled the close emotional bond they had with other primary attachment figures, such as their mothers. Some research suggests that the presence of a pet in the home provides not only a sense of physical safety and security, but can help people cope with symptoms of depression and anxiety due to stress (Cordaro, 2012; Doherty & Feeney, 2004; Sable, 1995; Watson & Weinstein, 1993). It is this strong and pervasive bond that makes grieving the loss of a pet sometimes as powerful and painful as the loss of another human. Since pets tend to have much shorter lifespans than people (with the exception of some birds and tortoises), pet loss is inevitable and grief is common. (For those species that may outlive their people, other problems may arise, such as on whom to bequeath guardianship of the pet after the death of the human.) Historically, acute grief after pet loss has been viewed as socially unacceptable, making it a "disenfranchised loss" (Packman et al., 2011). Today, more people are understanding of the unique pain of pet loss, yet it can still be dismissed by some as trivial. In this section, I will discuss the definition of a disenfranchised loss, the types and symptoms of grief due to pet loss, and suggestions for counseling clients who are grieving the death of a pet.

Grieving the Loss of a Pet

A disenfranchised loss is one that is not generally acknowledged or accepted by society (Attig, 2004). These are the types of loss that are socially not understood or are unsanctioned (Attig, 2004). Some examples of disenfranchised loss are the loss of a child by miscarriage or elective termination, the death of a lover in an extramarital affair, or the death of a pet (Lenhardt, 1997; Worden, 2008). Although these may seem like very different circumstances, they are similar in the sense that none are fully sanctioned by society as acceptable to mourn (Humphrey, 2009). The mourners often do not receive the social support of family and friends, and any public display of mourning may be perceived as strange or stigmatizing (Doka, 1989, 2002, 2008). In pet loss, it is common for other people to see the loss as superficial and expect the bereaved to quickly move on or to get a new pet (Packman et al., 2011). This expectation does not pay sufficient attention to the strength of the attachment formed between the person and their pet. When a pet loss is dismissed as trivial, it is based on the assumption that the relationship between a person and their pet is less profound than any relationship between humans. However, we now know that the connection between a person and their pet can be as deep and meaningful as relationships between humans, and pets are often viewed by humans as members of the family (Veldkamp, 2009). Since pets may provide a sense of nonjudgmental, unconditional love and support, the loss of a pet may be extremely painful, especially to those who do not have a strong support network. Stigmatization of public displays of mourning adds complication to grief in pet owners (Kaufman & Kaufman, 2006). Cordaro (2012) writes that "disenfranchised grief in the form of a socially unspeakable loss warns some pet owners that by society's norms, their genuine grief does not qualify for the empathy of a robust social support system" (p. 287). Therefore, the grieving pet owner is either socially stigmatized for their outward display of grief or feels forced to mourn in private, without any social support. To take one example of how such societal expectations are expressed, few companies allow bereavement time for those mourning the loss of a pet, although they often allow it for the loss of a human family member. Often pet loss ends up being a private, internalized grief, which may put the bereaved at a higher risk for a complicated or extended grief period.

Pet loss may also encompass anticipatory loss and ambiguous loss. Anticipatory loss is the feeling of grief that begins before the loss happens (Rolland, 1990). This is common with a prolonged illness, such as cancer. When a pet is diagnosed with a terminal illness, or is reaching an advanced age, the person must make difficult medical choices (sometimes limited by financial resources) and they may begin to grieve the loss of the pet before the pet's actual death; they mourn the pet as they were when healthy. Pet owners may also start thinking more about the upcoming death of their pet. Ambiguous loss also involves a loved one who has not died but is otherwise unavailable. The two types of ambiguous loss are when the loved one is alive but physically absent (such as when a pet is lost outside the home, stolen, or left behind due to a crisis incident) and when a loved one is physically present but psychologically absent, such as when a loved one suffers from a cognitive dysfunction like dementia (Boss, 2006). In any of these circumstances, the person may grieve the loss of the loved one as if they were dead, although they may technically still be alive; the grief is over the loss of the relationship as it once was. The difficulty with ambiguous loss is that the person is left without closure or, in some cases, even certainty about what has happened, and this may freeze the grieving process. The person may continue hoping to be reunited with the lost pet or searching for answers, thus delaying the grieving process, which may result in a more complicated form of grief (Boss, 2006). Ways to cope with an ambiguous loss include naming and acknowledging the feelings of loss, celebrating what remains of the relationship (the memories, etc.), and recognizing that some things are out of our control.

A disenfranchised loss may leave a person feeling as if their grief is insignificant (Attig, 2004), as people may say that the animal was "only a pet." When the disenfranchised loss is complicated by an anticipated or ambiguous loss, both internalized and externalized symptoms of grief can become amplified and complicate the grieving process (Cordaro, 2012; Lenhardt, 1997). Rather than isolate and stigmatize the bereaved pet owner, friends and family should be encouraged to empathize and support the person to aid the resolution of grief symptoms (Hall et al., 2004; Johansen, 1998).

Counseling for Pet Loss

One of the most important steps when counseling bereaved pet owners is to help them acknowledge the loss (Cordaro, 2012). This includes explaining the loss to children in a way they can understand. Since it is a loss that is not always recognized by society, it may feel as if the loss did not happen; in order to resolve grief symptoms, it is important to acknowledge the loss and associated feelings as real and valid. Clinicians can help the bereaved by using concrete language to describe the loss; words such as "death" and "dying" are less ambiguous than the figurative phrases "passed on" or "no longer with us." Psychoeducation is an important part of grief counseling. Clinicians should help the bereaved understand what constitutes a disenfranchised loss, internalized and externalized symptoms of grief, and that the grieving process neither has a set timeline nor is it linear. Group therapy for pet loss can be very helpful for the bereaved, since it normalizes the grief experience and allows the person to express their feelings in a nonjudgmental environment. Other grieving pet owners can also share mourning rituals and strategies that helped them cope. A favorite coping technique for pet loss is reading and sharing the *Rainbow Bridge* poems, works that explain death as a temporary state of being and describe how the pet will be patiently waiting, happy and healthy, to be reunited with their person over the rainbow bridge. The imagery underscores that the pet is no longer in pain, and provides hope that their separation is temporary. People with disorganized attachment styles and separation anxiety may especially benefit from any grief counseling that helps them understand that the relationship has not disappeared, even if the pet is no longer with them.

Clinicians may also suggest rituals to memorialize the pet, such as a funeral, memorial service, or the lighting of a candle. A pet funeral may seem odd to some people who don't understand the depth of the attachment bond, but a memorial service for a pet may help the bereaved achieve a sense of closure. Pet cemeteries and crematoriums often offer viewings which allow the pet owners to say their final goodbyes. Bereaved pet owners should also reach out to others who can help normalize and validate their feelings, such as online pet loss support groups on Facebook. In real life, the bereaved may feel rejected or misunderstood when they discuss their feelings of loss, but in a support group they may receive messages from hundreds of other bereaved pet owners who understand and normalize their pain. Just as in a traditional support group, these people may be able to provide coping strategies to help internalize the loss and aid in recovery.

Other strategies focus on making meaning out of the loss (Lichtenthal et al., 2010) through service: for example, helping others grieving a recent pet loss, volunteering at an animal shelter, donating to an animal charity, or publically sharing their story of pet loss. Turning grief into service creates meaning for the bereaved by helping them feel there was a purpose to the loss, and that something good can result out of a tragedy. In some cases, self-care techniques such as yoga or meditation can also assist in the processing of grief. Other coping techniques harness creativity: the bereaved might be encouraged to create a memorial altar or memory book, to write wishes for or messages to their pet on a piece of paper, or to practice journaling. Some people get a memorial tattoo of their pet, or wear a necklace that holds the pet's DNA, fur, or ashes. Although some people see pets as transitional objects in themselves, these wearable memories are transitional objects with respect to the bond with the pet. Like a favorite blanket may help a child feel closer to an attachment figure, wearable mementos help the bereaved feel that their connection to the deceased pet is more concrete and less ethereal (Winnicott, 1969).

I encourage people to speak to their pets as often as they would like in order to maintain this connection with their deceased pet for as long as they need it. However, clinicians should be aware of symptoms of prolonged or complicated grief, and in these cases they may want to stress the need for closure of the earthly relationship, despite an everlasting connection. Whether or not the grief is prolonged, I do not generally recommend that a client get another pet right away, since this may cause the client to suppress their loss rather than deal with it. It also may not be fair to the new pet if the client is so distraught that they are unable to form a bond with and adequately care for the new animal.

However, each person is different, and for some people the benefit from the apparent unconditional love and care provided by a support animal outweighs other considerations. It is important that the bereaved person understand the reasons why they are bringing a new pet into their home. Are they hoping to escape the pain of grief? Or do they feel that providing a loving home to a new pet will help them heal? It is also very important that clinicians are aware of the potentiality of suicidal thoughts, especially in those who view their pet as a primary support figure. In this case, suicide hotline information and information about the closest emergency room should be provided to the bereaved client.

Conclusion

The loss of a pet is similar to the loss of any close attachment figure or significant relationship in a person's life. As with grief over a human, a person grieving a pet may ruminate about how they could have saved their pet and what their pet would be doing if they were still alive (Cordaro, 2016). Yet it is still minimized by society, with people suggesting that the bereaved "get over it" since "it's just an animal." This attitude from the larger world makes pet loss a disenfranchised loss, in which people are made to feel that their loss is invalid or their emotional response is strange. A disenfranchised loss is more difficult to resolve, since the bereaved may not receive the same amount of social support as with other types of grief and loss. However, clinicians can suggest a number of coping strategies and resources to help the bereaved internalize the loss, accept a changed life without their beloved pet, and make meaning from the loss. Self-care is vitally important at this time, as is finding like-minded others who can validate the bereaved person's feelings. A clinician's validation and understanding of pet loss not only helps the bereaved, but may have wider-reaching effects, slowly changing societal norms and destigmatizing the pain of losing a pet.

Compassion Fatigue in the Veterinary Profession

Suicide

Suicide is the tenth leading cause of death in the United States (Hedegaard et al., 2020). In 2017, there were approximately 47,173 deaths by suicide in the United States and an additional estimated 1,400,000 suicide attempts (Centers for Disease Control and Prevention, 2018). Suicidal ideation is one of the major causes of psychiatric hospitalization, but it is often under-recognized and underreported. If a person does not notify others of his or her intent to end his or her life, the suicidal thoughts may go unnoticed until it is too late. Self-harm is only one of the potential warning signs of suicide, and in 2015 approximately 575,000 people visited a hospital for injuries due to self-harm (Centers for Disease Control and Prevention, 2018). However, though correlated, suicide and self-harm are separate phenomena, with many people who self-harm without the intention of completing suicide and others who complete suicide without first noticeably harming themselves.

As big a problem as suicide is, worldwide estimates suggest that veterinarians may have a four to six times higher suicide rate than the general population (Fink-Miller & Nestler, 2018; Milner et al., 2015; Tomasi et al., 2019). Although it is well-known that physicians, in general, are more prone than average to depression and suicidal ideation, there has been little information disseminated about suicidal ideation in the veterinary profession. United States Centers for Disease Control (CDC) figures show that, in the United States, female vets had a 3.5 times higher and male vets had a 2.1 times higher suicide rate than the general population (Centers for Disease Control and Prevention, 2018) (despite men overall completing suicide more frequently in the general population). By these estimates, veterinarians are twice as likely to complete suicide as other types of doctors or dentists (Fink-Miller & Nestler, 2018; Tomasi et al., 2019).

Although the CDC keeps a record of suicides by profession, to date little is known about the causes of suicide in the veterinary community. The purpose of this section is to highlight potential causes of suicide in veterinary professionals, the clinical implications of depression and suicidality in veterinarians, and the ways that clinicians can help reduce the number of veterinarian suicides.

Definitions

The veterinary profession appears to attract certain personality types that may cause them to be more prone to suicide (Allison, 2019; Fink-Miller & Nestler, 2018). For one, an integral part of the drive to become a veterinarian is a personality that has a highly developed sense of sympathy and empathy (Ayl, 2013; Fink-Miller & Nestler, 2018). Although these two terms appear interchangeable, they can be quite different. Sympathy is usually defined as experiencing similar views or emotions to another person (or nonhuman animal), whereas empathy is the capacity to see things from another's point of view and feel what they are feeling. We may describe sympathy as understanding another's viewpoint and empathy as putting yourself in the shoes of another.

Another important characteristic required of a veterinary professional is a deep sense of compassion (Ayl, 2013; Fink-Miller & Nestler, 2018). Compassion may be described as an understanding of the difficult situation of another to a point when you are moved to take action of some kind. Unfortunately, when a person feels compassion, sympathy, and empathy too often and in too overwhelming a manner, they may experience "compassion fatigue," a condition marked by mental fatigue, emotional distress, or apathy resulting from the constant demands of caring for others (Ayl, 2013; Figley & Roop, 2006). Burnout is another cluster of emotional, psychological, and physical reactions that result from feeling overwhelmed and unable to meet constant demands. In veterinarians, the stress and emotional strain of caring for others may cause compassion fatigue, while the logistical burden and constant daily demands of running a small business may cause burnout. Burnout also may cause a veterinarian to feel overwhelmed, exhausted, apathetic, and negative (Ayl, 2013).

Although there is a significant amount of stress and emotional strain involved in any helping profession, veterinarians are also susceptible to vicarious trauma (Ayl, 2013; Figley & Roop, 2006). As stated above, many veterinarians have a highly developed sense of empathy, and this is one possible cause for their vulnerability to emotional trauma. A vet may experience vicarious trauma when they view the trauma of their clients, resulting in PTSD-like symptoms that echo those of the client. Grief is a salient variable in veterinary work and, although it is a normal response to loss, experiencing it constantly as a result of vicarious trauma may cause a veterinarian painful emotions that push them toward wanting to end their life (Fink-Miller & Nestler, 2018).

Veterinary Medicine

The educational process for veterinarians is very rigorous, competitive, and expensive. It is often more difficult to get into veterinary school than medical school (there are fewer veterinary schools in the United States), but the cost of attending veterinary school is comparable (Ayl, 2013; Fink-Miller & Nestler, 2018). Veterinarians may therefore incur a large amount of student loan debt, but their annual income tends to be significantly lower than that of physicians treating humans (Allison, 2019; Centers for Disease Control and Prevention, 2018). They frequently work under stressful conditions with long hours, and they must have some business sense and manage staff and clients (Fink-Miller & Nestler, 2018). Finally, they must have access to lethal drugs and know how to be comfortable with frequently performing euthanasia, even in cases that may contradict their personal values (such as when an owner elects for euthanasia due to financial, not medical, reasons) (Allison, 2019; Nett et al., 2015; Tomasi et al., 2019). Research suggests that this combination of factors may be why veterinarians are especially vulnerable to suicidal ideation: they face burnout, deal with trauma, and have ready access to lethal means to complete suicide.

Notable Veterinarian Suicides

Some notable veterinarian deaths helped bring the issue of suicide among veterinarians to light. Dr. Sophia Yin was a 48-year-old, internationally known veterinary behaviorist (Kawczynska, 2014). She was well-established in the field as an author, philanthropist, scientist, and animal behaviorist (Kawczynska, 2014). Despite worldwide recognition and a highly successful career, on September 28, 2014 Dr. Sophia Yin was found hanged in her home, an apparent suicide (Kawczynska, 2014).

Clarissa Engstrom was a 44-year-old veterinarian and humanitarian who also took her own life, although unlike Dr. Yin, she used a lethal dose of pentobarbital, a medication commonly used in pet euthanasia (Coolican, 2012). Dr. Engstrom had worked extensively in animal behavior around the world, including rehabilitating baby chimpanzees in Zaire. When her work was stopped by political circumstances, she moved on to doing work with people suffering through the AIDS crisis. She had recently been arrested for an alleged vehicular incident but was released to her own home pending a trial. She never made it to court, since she was found dead in her home on May 21, 2012 (Coolican, 2012).

The story of Dr. Shirley Koshi is a cautionary tale about the dark side of veterinary medicine. Dr. Koshi had rescued a stray cat, provided it with veterinary care, and then kept it as her own pet (Mandlik & Larkin, 2014; Paddock & Marzulli, 2014). A woman appeared claiming that the stray cat belonged to her, since she fed it outside occasionally. When Dr. Koshi refused to return the cat to the streets, the woman filed a lawsuit and started a campaign of cyber-bullying Dr. Koshi, encouraging others to join in. The threats to the doctor became so severe that she had to close down her private practice because she was worried about her safety and the safety of her staff and clients (Mandlik & Larkin, 2014; Paddock & Marzulli, 2014). Although this appears to have been an extreme case, the rise in popularity of review sites such as Yelp has put business owners under increasing pressure to perform perfectly or risk receiving negative feedback, resulting in emotional distress and potential financial hardship. The financial burden of closing her practice was likely overwhelming to Dr. Koshi, and the lawsuit of the woman claiming the cat was undoubtedly stressful. Dr. Koshi completed suicide at 44 on February 16, 2014 by accute intoxication of phenobarbital, another drug commonly used in animal euthanasia (Mandlik & Larkin, 2014; Paddock & Marzulli, 2014).

Veterinarians and Suicide

There are few studies of suicidal ideation in veterinarians, but research shows that one in six vets has actively thought about suicide and approximately 66% of veterinarians currently suffer from depression, although to date the causes are not well defined (Centers for Disease Control and Prevention, 2018; Tomasi et al., 2019). The majority (75%) of veterinarians who completed suicide worked in a small animal practice (i.e., worked with dogs, cats, etc.), as opposed to those who worked with large animals (livestock), zoo animals, or exotic animals (Centers for Disease Control and Prevention, 2018). As in the general population, the majority of veterinarians who complete suicide use firearms as a means, but studies show that approximately 64% of female and 32% of male veterinarians who complete suicide—or 37% of the total—used self-poisoning as a means to end their life (Centers for Disease Control and Prevention, 2018). This would suggest that death by self-poisoning in the veterinary profession is 2.5 times more likely than in the general population (Centers for Disease Control and Prevention, 2018), possibly due to their easy access to and familiarity with administering lethal drugs. The CDC director, Dr. Robert Redfield, stated that "our findings suggest mortality from suicide among veterinarians has been high for some time—spanning the entire 36-year period we studied" (Centers for Disease Control and Prevention, 2018), and yet the high likelihood of veterinarian suicide is rarely discussed in the veterinary community or even among mental health professionals.

Risk Factors for Veterinary Suicide

What is it that makes veterinarians more likely to complete suicide than the average person? There are a number of variables at play in veterinarian suicide, including both internal and external factors (Ayl, 2013; Fink-Miller & Nestler, 2018). Internal factors include the neurological and psychological factors that make veterinarians great doctors. Veterinarians enter the field usually because of a desire to help animals, and although this desire may help them be a good vet, it is not always beneficial to them emotionally (Nett et al., 2015). An amplified sense of empathy and sensitivity to the suffering of others makes veterinarians especially vulnerable to the effect of mirror neurons, which are the neural basis for feelings of empathy (Ayl, 2013). Mirror neurons cause a repetition of feeling in the observer as demonstrated by the observed. When a veterinarian sees an animal suffering, in pain or discomfort, a highly empathetic personality makes them predisposed to feel that they, themselves, are also suffering, and the exposure is constant (Carmack, 2002; Figley & Roop, 2006; Fink-Miller & Nestler, 2018). These feelings may be compounded by witnessing the emotional suffering of animals' guardians when their pets are ill, injured, or dying (Compitus, 2019). Constant exposure to the pain and suffering of others makes vets especially susceptible to vicarious trauma and, eventually, compassion fatigue (Figley & Roop, 2006; Nett et al., 2015).

Other personality traits that help veterinarians to become successful doctors can make them more vulnerable to suicide and depression (Fink-Miller & Nestler, 2018). Vets are more likely to be overachievers and perfectionists (Ayl, 2013), traits that most likely helped them succeed in medical school but that may cause them to feel less self-compassion and become more self-critical than they would otherwise be (Crane et al., 2017). Finally, as with most helping professions, many veterinarians have difficulty saying "no" to others (Ayl, 2013). Many people in helping professions, such as social work, have difficulty maintaining boundaries because their desire to alleviate suffering is so strong (Compitus, 2019). But the lack of boundaries invites burnout and stress.

External factors that influence veterinarians' depression are time constraints and work-related stress (Ayl, 2013). Often veterinarians go into private practice and this practice can be isolating and also overwhelming (Fink-Miller & Nestler, 2018). They have limited access to peer support and have the burden of running a business by themselves (Larkin, 2018). There are few business classes in veterinary school, so many veterinarians learn on their own how to run a business. Vets must learn how to not just practice medicine, but manage staff and clients, oversee accounts and advertising, and administer other aspects of business (Fawcett, 2018; Larkin, 2018). They often work long hours, since most clients want appointments after work or on weekends. Some clients may also be difficult and/or demanding (Ayl, 2013), and may expect the veterinarian to charge a reduced fee or no fee because they know that the vet wants to help animals. Though most people would not think of haggling over the price at their own medical doctor, they are more likely to try to negotiate the price of veterinary care (Fawcett, 2018). If the vet complies too often, it may cause them additional financial difficulties. Compared with medical doctors, vets' training also offers a poor return on investment, since the price of veterinary school is as high as medical school and many vets have large student loan debt amounts, yet their salaries are usually significantly lower than that of a human medical doctor (Allison, 2019; Ayl, 2013). Vets may therefore have more difficulty paying back their student loans in comparison to their human doctor peers (Fink-Miller & Nestler, 2018). The average current student loan debt for a newly graduated veterinarian is over $143,000, but average starting pay is around $67,000 (Allison, 2019). The financial strain of running a business and/or having a large debt to pay off can easily add to depression.

Veterinarians enter the profession in order to help heal animals, but they may find themselves euthanizing animals more frequently than expected. The majority of veterinarians report that they would not become a vet again if they had the choice (Fink-Miller & Nestler, 2018; Crane et al., 2017). Vets are constantly exposed to death and dying, and yet are not taught how to process their own feelings of grief (few veterinary schools offer classes in self-care) (Ayl, 2013). As a veterinarian, they have access to deadly means (euthanasia drugs) and must be comfortable performing euthanasia frequently and for nonmedical reasons (financial, behavioral) (Ayl, 2013; Fink-Miller & Nestler, 2018). This combination of access to lethal means, the knowledge of how to administer the drugs, and the frequency with which veterinarians euthanize animals, creates a population that is particularly comfortable with man-made death as a means of escape, and that has the means to follow through on suicide. This is clearly a dangerous combination.

There are also external factors that emerge out of the internal struggles a vet may have. The constant exposure to death and grief may cause vicarious or secondary trauma, with pronounced PTSD symptoms, or even compassion fatigue (Figley & Roop, 2006). When a vet suffers from compassion fatigue, the resulting apathy may cause an exacerbation of the other factors in veterinary depression, such as a drop in client satisfaction (Fawcett, 2018; Figley & Roop, 2006). In a vicious circle, unhappy customers are likely to complain, the veterinarian may feel even more depressed, sad, hopeless, and helpless (Fawcett, 2018; Figley & Roop, 2006). In worst-case scenarios, the combination of social media and unhappy customers may result in cyber-bullying, which was likely the primary cause of Dr. Koshi's suicidal ideation (Allison, 2019; Mandlik & Larkin, 2014; Paddock & Marzulli, 2014). Possible additional factors in veterinary suicide include stigma around mental illness and a reluctance to attend therapy, poor job satisfaction, and a perceived inability to do their job properly (sadness about not being able to "save them all") (Figley & Roop, 2006).

Clinical Recommendations

Several steps can be taken to prevent veterinarians' depression from turning into suicidal ideation. We must reduce the stigma of therapy in the veterinary community (Kassem et al., 2019), as well as increase their access to mental health practitioners (Ayl, 2013; Larkin, 2018). Few veterinary schools currently offer classes on mental health, self-care, or wellness. Where these classes are offered, most are electives, and when faced with the option of choosing a mental health class or another medical class, trainee veterinarians are likely to choose the medical class over the self-care class. There is also limited information provided to veterinary students about the emotional burden of the profession (Larkin, 2018). We must increase access to mental health resources for veterinarians and normalize their experiences (Larkin, 2018).

Although there has been an increase in the number of veterinary social workers in veterinary hospitals, they are usually hired to support clients (i.e., pet guardians) and have limited time to support staff. Smaller vet clinics rarely have an in-house social worker. Linking mental health practitioners with veterinary schools would, perhaps, increase the number of veterinarians who seek out social workers for support. The social workers could also help the vets to identify emotional triggers in themselves, clients, and staff, and could teach them how to set boundaries with clients. The social workers could emphasize the need for self-care, including taking a vacation and self-reflection. Social workers could also teach adaptive coping techniques to veterinarians (journaling, listening to music, dancing, meditation, yoga, etc.).

In addition to working to bring such clinical social work services to veterinarians, we should increase the amount of research into compassion fatigue and depression in the veterinary community (Larkin, 2018). Even based on what we already know, there are numerous ways vets can be supported in the challenges they face. We must increase opportunities for vets to network and liaise with each other, as increasing the opportunities for socialization would reduce the chances of isolation (Kassem et al., 2018). Veterinarians should be encouraged to take business and management courses in order to increase their capabilities in this area of their field (Larkin, 2018). Social workers can also speak to vets about encouraging their clients to get pet insurance and to create pet wellness programs in order to save clients money (and increase client satisfaction) while still funding the veterinary clinic. Finally, clinicians can reach out to their own veterinarian friends and associates to see how social work services can be more easily integrated into a veterinary practice.

Current Initiatives

There currently is one nonprofit organization targeted specifically at preventing suicide completion in the veterinary community. Not One More Vet was developed in 2014 by Dr. Nicole McArthur to connect vets throughout the world and create an online support network (McArthur, n.d.). Because many veterinarians are working in private practice and may not have health insurance (due to high debt), Not One More Vet also offers financial assistance to vets who are unable to afford mental health treatment (McArthur, n.d.).

In 2018, the Royal College of Veterinary Surgeons (RCVS) in the United Kingdom and the American Veterinary Medical Association joined forces to promote Mind Matters, an initiative formed and funded by the RCVS in 2014 to address the high rate of completed veterinary suicides (Larkin, 2018). The purpose of Mind Matters is to increase support for veterinarians, reduce triggers, and reduce the stigma of seeking help for mental illness. Recent activities have included a campaign targeted at veterinarians to reduce the stigma of mental health counseling, training classes for vets in mindfulness meditation and self-care, a guide for managing stress in the workplace (for veterinary professionals), and a research symposium encouraging more research into suicide in the veterinary profession (Larkin, 2018).

Conclusion

The rate of completed suicide among veterinarians has remained high for the past few decades, yet it remains a well-hidden secret of the profession. Variables that influence veterinary depression include internal factors such as personality traits (perfectionists with high empathy) and the influence of mirror neurons, as well as external factors such as the constant exposure to grief and death, difficult clients, and limited knowledge about running a business (Ayl, 2013; Carmack, 2002). Veterinarians may also experience social isolation, financial difficulties, and limited access to mental health care (Allison, 2019; Kassem et al., 2019). They are at a high risk for compassion fatigue, secondary trauma, vicarious trauma, and even posttraumatic stress disorder (Ayl, 2013; Figley & Roop, 2006). With the rise of cyberbullying, veterinarians are vulnerable to attacks online, which may cause chronic emotional and financial distress (Allison, 2019). Most importantly, veterinarians have the knowledge and access to lethal means, and, as a job criterion, must be comfortable with causing death, and this makes them particularly susceptible to suicidal ideation (Allison, 2019). Mental health practitioners must be aware of the specific stressors of veterinary professionals in order to alleviate their symptoms of depression (Kassem et al., 2019). Mental health clinicians should reach out to veterinarians to normalize their experiences, and provide individual counseling and/or group counseling. The importance of self-care should not be overlooked, but these classes should be encouraged, or even required, in veterinary schools. Social workers should connect with these schools in order to facilitate a higher rate of participation in these classes. The rate of completed suicide among veterinarians can be reduced if we work together to reduce the stigma of mental illness and increase vets' access to mental health care.

References

Allison, L. (2019, April 9). *Veterinarian suicide rate at alarming level*. Retrieved from https://www.newsmax.com/health/health-news/veterinarian-suicides-suicides-veterinarians/2019/04/09/id/910820/

Attig, T. (2004). Disenfranchised grief revisited: Discounting hope and love. *Omega, 49*, 197–215.

Ayl, K. (2013). *When helping hurts: Compassion fatigue in the veterinary care professional*. AAHA Press.

Boss, P. (2006). *Loss, trauma, and resilience: Therapeutic work with ambiguous loss*. W. W. Norton & Company.

Carmack, B. J. (2002). *Grieving the death of a pet*. Augsburg Books.

Centers for Disease Control and Prevention. (2018, December). *New study finds higher than expected number of suicide deaths among U.S. veterinarians* (Press Release). Retrieved from https://www.cdc.gov/media/releases/2018/p1220-veterinarians-suicide.html

Cohen, S. P. (2002). Can pets function as family members? *Western Journal of Nursing Research. Special Issue: Human-Animal Interaction, 24*, 621–638. https://doi.org/10.1177/019394502320555386

Compitus, K. (2019). Traumatic pet loss and the integration of attachment-based animal assisted therapy. *Journal of Psychotherapy Integration, 29*(2), 119.

Coolican, J. P. (2012, May 21). *In remembering Dr. Clarissa Engstrom, friends and family will mobilize efforts against suicide*. Retrieved from https://lasvegassun.com/news/2012/may/21/remembering-dr-clarissa-engstrom-friends-and-famil/

Cordaro, M. (2012). Pet loss and disenfranchised grief: Implications for mental health counseling practice. *Journal of Mental Health Counseling, 34*(4), 283–294.

Crane, M. F., Phillips, J. K., & Karin, E. (2017). I've been a long time leaving: The role of limited skill transferability in increasing suicide-related cognitions and behavior in veterinarians. *Suicide and Life-threatening Behavior, 47*(3), 309–320.

Doherty, N. A., & Feeney, J. A. (2004). The composition of attachment networks throughout the adult years. *Personal Relationships*, 469–488. https://doi.org/10.1111/j.1475-6811.2004.00093.x
Doka, K. (1989). *Disenfranchised grief: Recognizing hidden sorrow*. Lexington Books.
Doka, K. (2002). *Disenfranchised grief: New challenges, directions, and strategies for practice*. Research Press.
Doka, K. (2008). Disenfranchised grief in a historical and cultural perspective. In M. S. Stroebe, R. O. Hansson, H. Schut, & W. Stroebe (Eds.), *Handbook of bereavement research and practice: Advances in theory and intervention* (pp. 223–240). American Psychological Association.
Fawcett, A. (2018). What do clients want in a veterinarian? *Veterinary Record, 183*(17), 531–533.
Figley, C. R., & Roop, R. G. (2006). *Compassion fatigue in the animal-care community*. Humane Society Press.
Fink-Miller, E. L., & Nestler, L. M. (2018). Suicide in physicians and veterinarians: Risk factors and theories. *Current Opinion in Psychology, 22*, 23–26.
Hall, M. J., Ng, A., Ursano, R. J., Holloway, H., Fullerton, C., & Casper, J. (2004). Psychological impact of the animal-human bond in disaster preparedness and response. *Journal of Psychiatric Practice, 10*, 368–374.
Hedegaard, H., Curtin, S. C., & Warner, M. (2020). Increase in suicide mortality in the United States, 1999–2018. *NCHS Data Brief, 362*, 1–8.
Humphrey, K. M. (2009). *Counseling strategies for loss and grief*. American Counseling Association.
Johansen, B. B. (1998). Care of the dying adolescent and the bereaved family. *Loss, Grief and Care, 2*, 59–67.
Kassem, A. M., Witte, T. K., Nett, R. J., & Carter, K. K. (2019). Characteristics associated with negative attitudes toward mental illness among US veterinarians. *Journal of the American Veterinary Medical Association, 254*(8), 979–985.
Kaufman, K. R., & Kaufman, N. D. (2006). And then the dog died. *Death Studies, 30*, 61–76. https://doi.org/10.1080/07481180500348811
Kawczynska, C. (2014, December). *Remembering Dr. Sophia Yin*. Retrieved from https://thebark.com/content/remembering-dr-sophia-yin
Kurdek, L. A. (2008). Pet dogs as attachment figures. *Journal of Social and Personal Relationships, 25*, 247–266. https://doi.org/10.1177/0265407507087958
Larkin, M. (2018). Taking mental health in a positive direction: U.K. vets work with AVMA to promote a culture change in the veterinary profession. *Journal of the American Veterinary Medical Association, 253*(8), 954–957.
Lenhardt, A. (1997). Grieving disenfranchised losses: Background and strategies for counselors. *Journal of Humanistic Education and Development, 35*, 208–216.
Lichtenthal, W. G., Currier, J. M., Neimeyer, R. A., & Keesee, N. J. (2010). Sense and significance: A mixed methods examination of meaning making after the loss of one's child. *Journal of Clinical Psychology, 66*(7), 791–812.
Mandlik, R., & Larkin, M. (2014, November 15). *Fighting the cyberbully*. Retrieved from https://www.avma.org/News/JAVMANews/Pages/141115a.aspx
McArthur, N. (n.d.). *Not one more vet*. Retrieved from: https://www.nomv.org/
Milner, A. J., Niven, H., Page, K., & LaMontagne, A. D. (2015). Suicide in veterinarians and veterinary nurses in Australia: 2001–2012. *Australian Veterinary Journal, 93*(9), 308–310.
Nett, R. J., Witte, T. K., Holzbauer, S. M., Elchos, B. L., Campagnolo, E. R., Musgrave, K. J., Carter, K. K., Kurkjian, K. M., Vanicek, C. F., O'Leary, D. R., Pride, K. R., & Pride, K. R. (2015). Risk factors for suicide, attitudes toward mental illness, and practice-related stressors among US veterinarians. *Journal of the American Veterinary Medical Association, 247*(8), 945–955.
Packman, W., Field, N. P., Carmack, B. J., & Ronen, R. (2011). Continuing bonds and psychosocial adjustment in pet loss. *Journal of Loss and Trauma, 16*(4), 341–357.
Paddock, B., & Marzulli, J. (2014, February 26). *New York veterinarian driven to suicide after cat custody battle ruins clinic*. Retrieved from https://www.avma.org/News/JAVMANews/Pages/141115a.aspx

Raup, D. G. (1999). Treasuring, trashing, or terrorizing: Adult outcomes of childhood socialization about companion animals. *Society & Animals, 7*, 141–159.

Rolland, J. S. (1990). Anticipatory loss: A family systems developmental framework. *Family Process, 29*(3), 229–244.

Sable, R. (1995). Pets, attachment, and well-being across the life cycle. *Social Work, 40*, 334–341.

Tomasi, S. E., Fechter-Leggett, E. D., Edwards, N. T., Reddish, A. D., Crosby, A. E., & Nett, R. J. (2019). Suicide among veterinarians in the United States from 1979 through 2015. *Journal of the American Veterinary Medical Association, 254*(1), 104–112.

Veldkamp, E. (2009). The emergence of "pets as family" and the socio-historical development of pet funerals in Japan. *Anthrozoös, 22*, 333–346.

Watson, N. L., & Weinstein, M. (1993). Pet ownership in relation to depression, anxiety, and anger in working women. *Anthrozoos: A Multidisciplinary Journal of The Interactions of People & Animals, 6*, 135–138.

Winnicott, D. (1969). The use of an object. *Internal Journal of Psycho-Analysis, 50*, 711–716.

Worden, J. W. (2008). *Grief counseling and grief therapy: A handbook for the mental health practitioner* (4th ed.). Springer.

Chapter 6
Crisis Intervention and the Human–Animal Bond

This chapter looks at the various types of crisis intervention services specifically designed for people with pets. I will define *people in crisis* as those who are without the basic needs as defined by Maslow (Abulof, 2017), including physiological needs (such as shelter), safety needs (such as personal security, resources, property), and love and belonging needs (such as family and sense of connection). The most important thing to note about people with pets in crisis is that by making them choose between their pets and the provision of services, we effectively prevent the people from attaining the most basic needs in Maslow's hierarchy, much less higher-level needs such as self-esteem, a sense of connection, and self-actualization (Abulof, 2017).

I start the chapter with a discussion of the significant number of people who are undomiciled (without a traditional home) and have pets as beloved family members. There is a major gap in service when it comes to this particular population, since the human–animal bond is often neglected when human basic needs are in jeopardy. In addition, there is some debate among animal welfare advocates over whether it is in the best interests of pets to live with people who do not have stable housing. The benefits and problems associated with pet guardianship for people in crisis are analyzed and discussed in this chapter. A large portion of the chapter focuses on the undomiciled; this is because many of the problems that this particular population faces are also present for other people with pets who are in crisis. Other types of crisis intervention involving the human–animal bond (HAB) are then discussed, such as people with pets in natural disasters, people with pets in domestic violence situations, and the effect of breed-specific legislation (especially with regard to systemic racism). Of course, attachment styles are considered within this discussion as an important aspect of pet guardianship. This chapter considers pet guardianship not just from an animal welfare perspective but through a social justice lens. Suggestions to help manage the well-being and health of people with pets who are in crisis are provided.

K. Compitus, *The Human-Animal Bond in Clinical Social Work Practice*, Essential Clinical Social Work Series,
https://doi.org/10.1007/978-3-030-87783-5_6

Homelessness

Even though most shelters and temporary housing do not allow pets, studies show that up to 24% of people without homes in the United States have companion animals (Irvine, 2013a). It is difficult to estimate the exact number of people without homes who are animal guardians, because many of these people are secretive about their pets; they are worried that their pets will be removed from them if they are found out (Irvine, 2013a). In addition, most of these people are not registered with local shelters, because there are very few shelters for the homeless that allow pets. Many animal guardians chose to live on the streets rather than give up their pet.

Pet guardianship can be expensive and there are few financial resources for people with pets. Some US states allow pet food to be purchased as part of public assistance, but many states do not. This means that to feed their pet, many people with limited incomes must choose to go hungry (Kidd & Kidd, 1994; Irvine, 2013b). There are few financial resources for veterinary care for pets of people with limited incomes, and usually these funds are only provided for emergency veterinary care and after an extensive application process. Not only are pets not allowed in housing, but they are often not allowed in stores, in hospitals/medical facilities, or on public transportation. This means that unless a homeless person has an existing support network, they often find it difficult to access medical care, since they have no one to care for their pet while they are at the doctor. Thus, many homeless people will forgo their own medical needs in order to remain with their pet (Howe & Easterbrook, 2018). This suggests that the limitations imposed on homeless pet owners by society often causes undue hardship, restricting access to services for the people.

Benefits of Pet Companionship for the Undomiciled

Research shows multiple benefits of pet guardianship, including lowered cholesterol, blood pressure, and lower chance of coronary artery disease (Beetz et al., 2012; Knight & Edwards, 2008; O'Haire, 2010). There are additional benefits to pet ownership for those who are without a home. Hutton (2015) found that the consistent care and companionship provided by pets are a steady source of support for the homeless. The bond that is formed when a homeless person cares for their pet may be considered an adaptive coping technique that helps alleviate social isolation and stigma, and may prevent depression (Hutton, 2015). Therefore, it is not surprising that researchers have found that people without homes often have especially strong attachment to their pets (Irvine, 2013b; Cronley et al., 2009). Irvine (2013b) found that "homeless men and women had significantly higher attachment scores than did those in the standardization group (the domiciled), with homeless men scoring higher than women" (p. 10).

There are various reasons why pets are such an important source of support in the lives of homeless people. Caring for their pet may provide a homeless person with a routine, a more structured day, and a sense of purpose. Many homeless people feel socially marginalized and stigmatized by the domiciled, and may view their pets as a nonjudgmental source of support (Compitus, 2019; Hutton, 2015). Like those who are domiciled, homeless people often describe their pets as family members or best friends. However, the homeless often also describe their connection with their pet as the only consistent social relationship in their lives, and aver that this is their only consistent love object and/or secure base (Kidd & Kidd, 1994). When interviewing street youth, Bender et al. (2007) found that "pets were identified as the youths' first priorities and were their companions, protectors, and sources of comfort. For many street youth, who had little connection to their biological family, pets were described as the 'closest thing you have to kin out there'" (p. 33). The bond is often so strong that some individuals report that preserving their bond with their pet is their primary goal in life and the basis for all other life decisions (Cronley et al., 2009).

As attachment objects and the alleviators of social isolation, the pets of the homeless are vital to preventing their guardians' loneliness (Irvine, 2013b; Rew, 2000). Pets can also be considered vehicles of redemption and provide a purpose for living. They encourage a sense of responsibility in the person and "the animal's dependence offers immediate ways to express care, allowing for the manifestation of a 'good' self. The fulfillment of the associated responsibilities requires a sacrifice, which, in these stories, involves giving up drugs and alcohol or deciding to live in the car" (Irvine, 2013b, p. 22). Thus, the pets are not only vehicles of redemption, but witnesses to the personal narrative of the person's struggles. Irvine et al. (2012) write that "the activities of taking care of a pet help justify a positive sense of self, especially among those who have few resources to spare" (p. 28). They help the person form a stronger sense of self-worth, while loving without judgment.

The connection between a homeless person and their pets, and the sense of responsibility they feel to care for their pets, may be so strong as to help resolve many psychosocial stressors. Pets may alleviate loneliness and depression, and can help prevent suicide (Rew, 2000). This may even result in lower levels of criminal activity (Rew, 2000; Irvine, 2013b; Taylor et al., 2004), since the homeless person who does not want to lose their pet may be less likely to risk going to jail. Baker (2001) found that homeless people with dogs are also less likely to use drugs than those who do not have dogs (Irvine, 2013b). Pets may provide the homeless with an increased sense of personal security; this is especially true of homeless women, many of whom are homeless as a result of leaving a domestic violence situation (Cronley et al., 2009).

Limitations of Pet Ownership

Although there are many benefits to having a pet while homeless, there are aspects of homelessness that may make it difficult to keep a pet. Although animals are a constant source of companionship for homeless people, their pets are usually not allowed into buildings or private facilities. This means that a homeless person may not be able to enter a soup kitchen to get a meal, or a shelter to take a shower, since their pet is not allowed in these buildings (Irvine, 2013b). If the pet owner desired to enter the building, they would first have to secure a trusted person to watch their pet while they were inside. Often those with pets are dependent on their companion animal because they do not have close relationships with other humans, so securing a pet sitter, even for a few minutes, may be difficult (Baker, 2001; Irvine, 2013b). In fact, those with pets are more socially isolated (sometimes because they only trust their pet), and perhaps the stress of finding pet care in an emergency is one of the reasons that homeless people with pets are more likely to suffer from panic attacks than those without pets (Baker, 2001; Irvine, 2016).

Taylor et al. (2004) found that homeless people with pets had lower health scores, primarily due to a lack of access to facilities that allowed their pets. They found that, because the pet was not allowed inside medical facilities, and often there was nobody else to care for the pets, homeless pet owners were significantly less likely to use medical facilities than those without pets (Taylor et al., 2004; Irvine, 2016). Baker also found that "twice as many [pet] owners as non-owners suffered from mental health and social issues, such as anxiety, aggressive behavior, and isolation" (Baker, 2001; Irvine, 2013b, p. 10), although it was not determined whether the mental health issues existed before pet ownership and whether or not pet ownership alleviated these behavioral symptoms.

Since their pets are such an important attachment figure for the homeless, Singer et al. (1995) found that homeless people with pets are very likely to refuse housing if they cannot bring their pet with them. This is a bit of a conundrum, since most shelters, hostels, and rentals do not allow pets (Baker, 2001) and a large majority of homeless people with pets have been denied housing as a result of pet ownership (Singer et al., 1995). These people are, therefore, left to find their own forms of shelter, and sheltering in untraditional places may have repercussive effects. Some studies reflect a higher number of homeless people with pets having a problem with alcohol (Baker, 2001); this may be a maladaptive coping technique that has developed among those unable to avail of shelter, due to the warming effects of alcoholic liquids.

Some researchers hypothesize that people with pets may remain homeless longer due to pet ownership, since they have a more difficult time securing permanent housing that allows their pet (Singer et al., 1995). Labrecque and Walsh (2011) found that those homeless people who relinquished their pets "in exchange for shelter spoke of the pain, trauma, and negative effects that relinquishing a pet had on themselves and their children" (Irvine, 2016, p. 11). Since there are many homeless people who continue to live on the streets with their pets, it can be inferred that, at least in subjective terms, the benefits to pet ownership may greatly outweigh the negative aspects of living on the street (Irvine, 2016).

Animal Welfare

To the casual observer, a homeless person with a pet may appear unable to care for the basic needs of the pet. However, Irvine reported that "the animals I observed were in reasonably good health, although a few had serious issues such as cancer that were most likely unrelated to their living situation" (Irvine, 2013b, p. 30). It is well known that many homeless people, cognizant that their dogs are dependent on them as caretakers, feed their pets first, even if that means that they will go hungry themselves. These people know that if their pet was not with them, the pet would likely be sent to a shelter and euthanized due to overcrowding. Therefore, the sacrifices that homeless people make to care for their pets may help them to feel redeemable and worthy, and caring for their pet may provide them with a sense of meaning.

Some homeless people argue that the way the domiciled care for pets may actually be more immoral and unethical; they cite long days alone at home as poor animal welfare, while the pets of the homeless are rarely, if ever, left alone (Irvine, 2016). They cite the constant companionship between the pets and people as a healthy source of social support for both the person and the animals. Homeless people reported that they were more likely to seek medical care for their pets than for themselves and that the health and well-being of their pets was a top priority (Cronley et al., 2009). The constant focus on the pet as a vehicle of redemption, and placing the needs of the pets before their own, demonstrates that the welfare of their pets is a primary focus of most homeless pet guardians, even if their pets must live with them in untraditional locations.

Social Justice Lens

Irvine et al. (2012) report that homelessness is one of the most stigmatized conditions in the modern world and being homeless with a pet can make the person even more subjected to judgment by strangers. It is fairly common for homeless people with pets to be confronted by strangers and accused of not having the best interests of the animal in mind (Irvine et al., 2012). However, some kind strangers may understand the additional psychosocial stressors of a homeless person with pets, and may be more likely to donate money, pet food, or pet supplies to the homeless pet owner than to one without a pet.

Despite a worldwide interest in human rights, the rights of the homeless are often overlooked in general (Sen, 2004), and those of the homeless with pets are greatly neglected. Primarily, it is the right of a homeless person to have an animal companion as they see fit. However, Sen writes that some critics "propose a discriminating rejection: they accept the general idea of human rights but exclude, from the acceptable list, specific classes of proposed rights, in particular the so-called economic and social rights, or welfare rights" (p. 316). There are those who may suggest that the homeless have basic rights, such as the right to shelter or food, but then state that pet ownership is not a basic human right and, therefore, should not be protected by welfare laws (Rhoades et al., 2015). Though the United Nations' Universal Declaration of Human Rights, drafted in large part by Eleanor Roosevelt, states that "all are equal before the law and are entitled without any discrimination to equal protection of the law" (Art. 6), homeless people with pets are not allowed the same access to services as those without pets. The law may be nondiscriminatory in its formulation, but many social policies continue to discriminate in effect based on certain dimensions of a person's life.

We have seen that caring for a pet can help foster a positive sense of self, a sense of worth, and a motivation for remaining sober and out of jail; there is no doubt that companion animals provide a stable sense of support and a nonjudgmental source of affection, and are vehicles of redemption. In these roles they feed the basic psychological needs of the homeless, the need to feel loved and a reason to love themselves. And yet advocacy for human rights, as a social justice cause, generally attends to social freedoms only as they apply to human-to-human social connections. Pets are not allowed in shelters, yet the homeless with pets deserve shelter, and also to be able to maintain their pets as valid sources of support. Since pet owners consider their pets as family, they should be allowed to keep their "family" with them when they seek shelter or medical care. If the pets are not allowed inside it means that the shelter system is inadequate, discriminatory, and only set up to address the needs of homeless people without pets. Lawmakers, therefore, should consider reformation of the policies governing homeless shelters as essential. As Sen writes, "the current unrealizability of any accepted human right, which can be promoted through institutional or political change, does not, by itself, convert that claim into a non-right" (Sen, 2004, p. 320). Just because pet ownership is considered by many to be a luxury, not a right, does not mean that owning a pet is not a right. If a pet provides emotional support to a person, how can we say that that person has to choose between keeping warm inside or keeping happy outside with their pet?

Perhaps it is their membership in a different subgroup that causes homeless people with pets to be further marginalized by society (Catala, 2015). Irvine (2013b) explains that, similar to Rawlsian justice, "pet ownership is considered nearly a birthright in contemporary Western societies. In most people's everyday lives, the right to animal companionship and the ability to provide care go uncontested. The homeless are likely the only group criticized and stigmatized for having pets" (p. 49). Homeless youth with pets, in particular, are known to be stigmatized by society and are often, surprisingly, rejected by those who should be helping them, such as police officers and case managers (Bender et al., 2007).

Banerjee (2005) considers whether those who earn a wage are considered more deserving of social justice. Homeless people with pets are unable to leave their pets alone, making it harder for them to pursue full-time jobs. In turn, this inability to work may be seen as a lack of motivation to work, and sign of a lower moral worth than those who are or can work. But placing the needs of their pets before their own, and not working so that they can care for their pets, is not equivalent to a lack of motivation to work (Banerjee, 2005). Rather, it illustrates a concern for others, specifically for innocents, that should be commended and not condemned. Banerjee (2005) suggests that, rather than judging people by our own needs, we should allow others to "define their own situations and contribute to the development and evaluation of solutions" (p. 38). The involvement of people in creating a solution to their problems is likely to result in more successful programs, and also gives participants a sense of ownership over their work. Sadly, brainstorming multiple ways for the homeless with pets to access services is not considered a priority to most lawmakers.

The Universal Declaration of Human Rights also states that "no one shall be subjected to arbitrary arrest, detention or exile" (Art. 9) and that "no one shall be subjected to arbitrary interference with his privacy, family, home or correspondence, nor to attacks upon his honour and reputation" (Art. 12). However, homeless people with pets have been effectively exiled from medical centers and shelters, since they are unable to leave their pets alone. Despite the human rights declaration, they are continuously subjected to arbitrary interference with their family because they are asked to leave their pets outside, unattended and vulnerable, perhaps to suffer or die, if they are to have their basic needs filled. The homeless with pets are attacked, as mentioned above, by those who believe that they have no right to keep an animal with them, since some onlookers believe that they are unable to care for themselves. The treatment the homeless with pets endure is, therefore, in direct violation of the declaration of rights, yet this is a subject that is not often discussed as a matter of importance. People are being asked to choose between their "family" and getting food, medical care, or shelter from storms, an impossible choice to ask anyone. These are basic rights that anyone deserves, regardless of whether their family is a human or nonhuman animal. And yet, according to Rawlsian justice, fair access is not the same as equal access; as long as people are technically free to access services, they are receiving just treatment (Banerjee, 2005). In Rawlsian justice, pet ownership is a luxury, not a necessity, and therefore inconsequential. However, for the homeless person with a pet, that animal is not in any sense a luxury. Their companion animal is their secure base, their family, and a source of emotional stability; abandoning that animal is not an option.

We know that there are numerous physiological and psychological benefits to pet ownership. Therefore, agencies that serve the homeless, rather than turning away pet guardians, should consider incorporating pets into their programs. Sadly, "the failure to accommodate the needs of pet owners can deter some from seeking services (Kidd & Kidd, 1994) or force them to relinquish their pets in exchange for shelter" (Labrecque & Walsh, 2011, p. 84). As mentioned above, the effects of relinquishing an animal can be seriously detrimental to the homeless person's emotional state and is not recommended for anyone. Given that homeless shelters are notorious for being dangerous, it is likely that some pet owners also feel safer in the shelter system when they are allowed to keep their pet with them, as a physical and psychological source of protection (Rhoades et al., 2015). Therefore, there is a strong need for pet-friendly housing, shelters, soup kitchens, and medical facilities, all of which would allow people to maintain their connection to their pet.

It is important to note that studies show few people have lost their housing due to pet ownership, but that pet ownership is a significant barrier to reestablishing housing (Baker, 2001; Irvine, 2013b, p. 11). Those who are homeless with pets are not always single adults. This demographic includes unaccompanied youth, families with or without children, and those escaping domestic violence. There are a wide variety of people who may end up homeless and may seek the comfort of a pet. To marginalize, stigmatize, and refuse services to these people is a true violation of their human rights.

Future Directions

Homeless pet owners describe how important it is to keep their pets with them, regardless of the implications for meeting their own basic needs (Bender et al., 2007). In fact, studies show that "61% of acutely and 93% of chronically homeless individuals with animals wished to find housing, but 96% of acutely homeless and 93% of the chronically homeless individuals said they would never live without their animals" (Singer et al., 1995, p. 856). This suggests that it is vitally important to pay attention to policies that ban (or allow) pets when providing services to this population (Cronley et al., 2009). We need a paradigm shift, whereby homeless people's relationships with their animals come to be seen as signs of strength: such relationships represent an adaptive coping technique for the stressors of being homeless, having medical problems, or facing financial and food insecurity. They have found a way to feel good about themselves despite adverse life events. They have redefined companion animal guardianship as something that reflects their inner character and provides meaning to their lives. They may begin to see themselves as capable of caring for another, rather than helpless and at the mercy of society (Irvine et al., 2012). Pet ownership may then give them a sense of control in a world where they otherwise feel little control over their state of being. Providing care for another may, in turn, causes a change in personal identity, and the homeless person may see themselves as a good person, rather than a societal reject (Irvine et al., 2012).

The first step in making a change is for all organizations that serve the homeless (whether medical clinics, hospitals, soup kitchens, or shelters) to develop policies that recognize the role of pets in clients' lives. This will include intake forms that ask in detail about pet ownership and explore the meaning of that relationship with the client. If the agencies are not able to house the pets within their walls, they should develop connections with animal care agencies that can assist in temporary care of the animal while the person receives services. It is also important to offer housing referrals that allow pets, since those with pets are likely to reject any housing option that does not accommodate them. Finally, Graham (2019) writes that "the potential differences in housing needs among pet owners experiencing homelessness and those housed into the rental market should not detract from the main implication in reviewing this literature, which is that pet owners need more options for affordable, safe, and accessible housing. As well, pet owners need support and assistance to navigate housing transitions. The failure to accommodate pets in housing is a moral issue for society at large, not least because of the detrimental impacts that pet loss can have on the well-being of both human and animal populations" (p. 28).

Domestic Violence

No less important than those without homes are those who are living in a home filled with fear. According to the National Domestic Violence Hotline (n.d.), "more than 1 in 3 women and 1 in 4 men in the U.S. will experience rape, physical violence, and/or stalking by an intimate partner." There certainly are social service agencies, such as the National Coalition Against Violence and the National Domestic Violence Hotline, that provide resources for people who are fleeing an abusive partner. However, up to 48% of domestic violence victims hesitate to escape their abusers because they are concerned about what will happen to their pets when they leave (Haden et al., 2018). The majority of resources for victims of intimate partner violence (IPV) do not include resources for people with pets. As discussed in previous chapters, many people view their pets as beloved family members, akin to a child, buddy, or best friend. However, when it comes to domestic violence (DV), the majority of DV shelters and safe spaces do not allow people to bring their pets. It is understandable that the shelters want to focus their resources on helping the people escaping violent partners. However, 71% of pet-owning women entering women's shelters reported that their batterer had injured, maimed, killed, or threatened family pets as revenge or to psychologically control victims; 32% reported their children had hurt or killed animals (Wood et al., 1997). Asking these already vulnerable people to leave a furry family member behind is often adding another layer of trauma to an already traumatic situation. Those who enter a domestic violence shelter are asked to choose between their own life and that of their beloved pet; 52% of victims in shelters have no choice but to leave their pets behind with their batterers (Wood et al., 1997).

Why should clinical social workers consider the pets of people in IPV situations? Typically, domestic abusers tend to isolate their victims from other friends and family. Often, the victim's pet becomes the only source of emotional support and unconditional love that the victim may have. Studies reveal that approximately 18–48% of women entering shelters delayed their escape due to concerns for the welfare of pets or even livestock left behind. Often, people who abuse their partner report harming the family pets first because it is less likely to get the attention of police (Newberry, 2017). Abusers may also harm the pets out of jealousy of the emotional connection between the animal and the partner, or as a form of threatening their intended target (e.g., hitting the family dog as an example of how the abuser is planning to hit their spouse) (Stevenson et al., 2018). Of course, it is well established that animal abusers often "graduate" from violence toward animals to violence toward humans, and one of the indicators for antisocial personality disorder (psychopathy) is violence toward animals (Hansen, 2020). A strong connection has been established between violence toward animals and other antisocial behavior, including drug offenses and other criminal behavior (such as stealing and public brawls, etc.). However, the temporal order in which these offenses occur varies; animal abuse may precede violence against humans or other criminal behavior, or vice versa (Newberry, 2017).

What is established is that many victims of IPV remain in the relationship because they do not want to leave their pet behind and they feel that they have no other option (Strand & Faver, 2006). There are less than 3000 shelters for abused women, men, and children, and less than 3% of these can accommodate pets (Strauss & Brulliard, 2018). Of that 3%, most are not actually providing pet-friendly housing, but instead are partnering with local shelters and rescue groups to provide temporary boarding for the pets (Ascione, 2000); Red Rover is a national agency that aids DV survivors in securing local pet boarding for free or low rates. Although this option provides safe living for all, the victim and their pet are still separated and the victim's emotional healing is hampered by this arrangement. Of those rare facilities that can care for pets in-house, most have limited space for pets and can only accommodate one or two at a time. While these options allow victims and pets to escape abuse, the facilities' acceptance of such a limited number of pets misses the opportunity to tap into the power of the human–pet bond with a consciously created co-living environment conducive to healing.

The Urban Resource Institute in NYC is one of the first agencies that have created facilities to shelter IPV survivors along with their families and pets. Their program is called the PALS program (People and Animals Living Safely) and not only provides co-living spaces for people and their pets, but other resources for these families, such as pet supplies and pet food. Those who are in crisis are in a state of disequilibrium and it is important for them to feel safe and secure so that emotional healing can start. The housing of IPV survivors with their pets is vitally important because not only does it provide the person with a sense of normality, it also allows them to maintain their emotional support system and, as discussed previously, the presence of a beloved animal may also promote emotional and physical healing.

Disaster Relief

Hurricane Katrina was one of the deadliest natural disasters in the history of the United States (U.S. Senate, 2006). The category 5 hurricane caused approximately 1800 deaths and $125 billion dollars' worth of damage in New Orleans and the surrounding areas in August 2005 (Vigdor, 2008). One of the major problems that the hurricane caused was flooding in 80% of the city of New Orleans, which left tens of thousands of people without access to basic needs such as food and shelter and unable to escape or communicate their needs to others due to a damaged infrastructure (U.S. Senate, 2006).

In response to the hurricane, the White House and Department of Homeland Security (DHS) assessed the existing emergency response plans on both a local government and state levels and determined that all response plans should be integrated with the federal government in order to receive federal funding (Sobel & Leeson, 2006). The assessment stated specifically that "state and local evacuation plans should specify procedures to address the pre-positioning of food, medical, and fuel supplies. These plans should address establishing first-aid stations, tracking and coordinating movements of evacuees, evacuating pets, unaccompanied minors, the elderly, and evacuating people who lack the means to leave voluntarily" (United States, 2006).

This marked the first time that pets were included in government evacuation plans. It is estimated that during Hurricane Katrina alone, approximately 250,000 cats and dogs died or were displaced as a result of this lack of inclusion (Hunt et al., 2008). In addition, many people were forced to choose between saving their own lives and staying with their pet; some people refused to evacuate because they knew that they would have to abandon their pets as a result (Hunt et al., 2008). Other people were forced to evacuate and leave their furry family members behind, but the pain of leaving their pets to face near-certain death was an extremely distressing way to survive an already traumatic situation. Even those who managed to take their pets with them had more difficulties to surmount, since pets were usually not allowed in disaster relief shelters and pet supplies were not provided.

Due to the large number of people who reported extreme distress and traumatic symptoms as a result of the death or abandonment of their pets, in the fall of 2006 Congress passed the Pets Evacuation and Transportation Standards Act of 2006, also known as the PETS Act (H.R. 3858), which was signed into law by President Bush in October (United States, 2006). The PETS Act ensures that all local and state emergency plans include the needs of people with pets and service animals following a major disaster. The PETS Act gave primary responsibility for people with pets to the Federal Emergency Management Agency (FEMA) and states that FEMA is authorized to rescue, care, shelter, and provide essential needs for household animals during a major disaster (Edmonds & Cutter, 2008). PKEMRA (the Post-Katrina Emergency Management Reform Act) was later added to the PETS Act to expand the role of the federal agency by designating FEMA as responsible to ensure pet rescue and shelter and to liaise with partner agencies such as the Department of Agriculture, the Department of Health and Human Services (HHS), and the Red Cross (LaVoy, 2019).

Although the PETS act and PKEMRA were very necessary and well-intentioned policies, they were enacted too late to help thousands of people and pets during Hurricane Katrina. They also left some large gaps in service that did not come to light until Hurricane Maria struck Puerto Rico in 2017 (Parker, 2019). During Maria, many residents of Puerto Rico had their homes destroyed but were unable to leave the island with their pets (Parker, 2019). Unfortunately, FEMA and the PETS Act do not require that privately owned hotels or airplanes allow pets in the case of a national disaster. Many residents of Puerto Rico had their homes destroyed, but were unable to transport their pets to safety, thus causing thousands of pets to die due to abandonment, lack of food, or medical care during Hurricane Maria and the months that followed (Parker, 2019). The shelters in Puerto Rico were already overflowing with stray animals, but they then had to deal with a growing feral population, since those abandoned animals that survived the hurricane in many cases began living on the streets, where they reproduced.

Just as with Katrina, many families that survived Maria were unable to access the emotional support, care, and love of their pets in their time of need (Leonard & Scammon, 2007; Walsh, 2009). Instead, families who lost their homes, jobs, and human family members also often also had to grieve the loss of a pet. These natural disasters did not only affect those who already had fixed incomes, but also affected those in the middle class, since the limitations on pets in hotels or on airplanes affected people in crisis at most socioeconomic levels. Although these gaps in service have recently been brought more into the public awareness, we have yet to see any major public policy changes to address the missing resources.

Breed-Specific Legislation

Breed-specific legislation (BSL) are those laws that prevent people from having or maintaining certain breeds of dogs, regardless of the temperament of the individual dog. I have included BSL in this chapter on crisis intervention because I have personally worked with clients who have had to sleep in their cars or give up housing on the threat of having their cherished pet removed from their care, simply because their dog looks a certain way. Typically, BSL targets "Pit Bull-type" dogs, which are often described as dogs having a square-shaped head, or is a pure or mixed breed dog that includes any of the following breeds: American Pit Bull Terrier, American Staffordshire Terrier, Staffordshire Bull Terrier, Boxer, Dogo Argentino, American Bulldog, Boston Terrier, among others (Olson et al., 2015). Pit Bull-type dogs are banned in many cities in the United States including Miami, Denver, and St. Louis (Ledger et al., 2005). However, BSL also targets any breed of dog that is deemed "dangerous to the public" and may include Akitas, Mastiffs, and other breeds of dog—even Labrador Retrievers were almost banned in Toronto for the same reasons that Pit Bulls are banned today (Graham et al., 2019).

BSL is, therefore, a major cause of crisis and distress for many people and can increase a need for services, including housing. News articles over the past few years have highlighted the prejudice that people with Pit Bull-type dogs face, including the banning of their work as service dogs for autistic children (Campbell, 2009) and psychiatric service dogs for veterans with PTSD (Campbell, 2009). In her book *Pit Bull: The Battle over an American Icon*, Bronwen Dickey (2017) even describes BSL as potentially the result of systemic and institutionalized racism. She writes that as people of color gravitated toward Pit Bull-type dogs, BSL became more popular with landlords as a legal way of preventing people of color from moving into primarily white building complexes. As stated earlier, BSL is not limited to just Pit Bull-type dogs, and as breed preferences change, new legislation may give landlords the ability to add to their list of banned breeds.

There are several reasons why BSL is not only ineffective but also harmful to people with pets. First, a systemic analysis of dog attacks in the media has shown that a large number of dog attacks were misrepresented as being caused by a Pit Bull-type dog, when often this was not the case (Cohen & Richardson, 2002). The researchers hypothesized that the term "Pit Bull" would sensationalize a news item more than an accurate description of the dog; for example, if an English Bulldog attacked a person it would be deemed less newsworthy than if it was reported as a Pit Bull. The term "Pit Bull" has been demonized by the media and now conjures mental images of snarling, violent dogs, when most Pit Bull-type dogs are actually quite affectionate, goofy, and loving (Dickey, 2017; Lockwood & Rindy, 1987). In fact, the vast majority of dog attacks were from dogs that were very badly abused and taught to attack, and/or affected by human negligence/neglect, regardless of breed (Lockwood & Rindy, 1987). And yet, Pit Bulls are not allowed in many government-run housing facilities, such as the housing projects run by the NYC housing authority. If a Pit Bull-type dog is found, they are removed from the home and brought to the local shelter (often a kill shelter). It is extremely problematic and harmful to the mental health and well-being of a person who views their dog as a strong source of social support when a beloved family pet is removed from their home and destroyed just because of misinformation.

The "Pit Bull-type dog" category is so loosely defined, and encompasses so many different breeds that I often think of it as a new alternative to the word "mutt." Since there is no DNA test that will verify whether an animal is a "Pit Bull type," currently a dog can be removed from their home, seized by police, euthanized, or banned from cities, solely based on the shape of the dog's head and the idea that perhaps the dog may have an ancestor that was used for fighting. In truth, many of the breeds considered Pit Bull-type dogs were known as "Nanny Dogs" at the start of the twentieth century because of their affectionate nature, and it was common for people to have Pit Bull-type dogs watch over and care for their children (Dickey, 2017).

To be clear, there is one type of purebred dog, the American Pit Bull Terrier (ABPT), which can be identified in DNA tests (though the American Kennel Club does not recognize this as an official pure breed in the United States). The problem is that purebred dogs have standards: When we say "Labrador," for example, a standard image of a Labrador Retriever comes to mind. The breed clubs have set size, weight, and color requirements for each breed, to differentiate a purebred dog from a mixed-breed dog. However, when "Pit Bulls" are discussed in common parlance and in the media, this term can refer to a wide range of dogs that do not fit any standards. They come in all sizes (from 25 to 130 lbs), colors, and shapes, and there appears to be no common physical feature other than a square-shaped jaw. Therefore, the vast majority of dogs commonly labeled as Pit Bulls do not meet the breed standard for the ABPT as set by the international kennel clubs. Most also do not genetically match the ABPT, since the square head that justifies their inclusion in the "Pit Bull" category is due to being a descendant of another breed with a square-shaped head.

The sloppy categorization of Pit Bull-type dogs is only the beginning. There is a huge amount of misinformation about Pit Bull-type dogs, much of which is perpetrated by the media and by malicious websites. The idea of a "locking jaw" is one of the most well-known myths, despite the fact that it is completely biologically inaccurate and impossible. The idea that this giant population of mixed-breed dogs are all aggressive is also laughable. In fact, studies show that the ABPT and other Pit Bull-type breeds (American Staffordshire Terrier, etc.) score among the highest of all dog breeds when put through a temperament test (Cohen & Richardson, 2002); this signifies that they are some of the most well-tempered dogs that exist. In fact, Pit Bull-type dogs score higher on scores of good temperament than other popular breeds such as Yorkshire Terriers, Havanese, Poodles, and Portuguese Water Dogs (the preferred breed of former President Obama) (Cohen & Richardson, 2002). In studies of the prevalence of dog bites, Dachshunds and Chihuahuas consistently come in as the two breeds most likely to attack a human (Duffy et al., 2008).

Ironically, it is often the kindest and most loving dogs that end up being demonized; this is because those who are prone to abuse dogs tend to choose docile animals, and within this criterion have preferred breeds that change over time (Dickey, 2017). In the 1980s, it was the Doberman; in the 1990s, it was the Rottweiler; currently, it is the Pit Bull-type dog. All these dogs tend to have a naturally agreeable nature. They are then trained commonly as fighting dogs. The idea is to train them to attack another dog, not a human; however, when an animal is taught to fight it is never with kindness, and general aggression in the animal is the inevitable result (Bulgakov, 2013). Just as a horribly abused human may hurt others, any dog that is badly abused has the potential to harm someone, regardless of breed. Nonetheless, even abused animals can be redeemed; for example, many of the dogs that were violently abused by football player Michael Vick went on to become therapy dogs (Gorant, 2011). Once they were removed from the abusive situation and treated with loving kindness, their resilient nature allowed them to heal and return to a trusting relationship with humans.

Since those who abuse dogs and train them to fight are not interested in obeying the law, BSL in practice serves to limit the rights only of law-abiding citizens. Those who are already fighting and abusing dogs will continue to do so, regardless of any breed ban. In addition, if the abusers cannot access the banned breed, they will simply move on to abusing another breed of dog. BSL, therefore, does not stop animal abuse, nor does it stop the creation of fighting animals. It merely limits a pet owner's freedoms by dictating what their dog should look like, something that seems legally indefensible.

Sadly, the myths and lies about Pit Bull-type dogs have led to them being banned in many countries throughout the world without just cause. Some home insurance companies even charge a higher or lower premium, depending on the type of dog you have (Cohen & Richardson, 2002), without cause or proof that the dog is a nuisance. BSL, therefore, severely limits human rights, costs law-abiding citizens more money, and wastes the time and money of any local government, while doing nothing to stop those who abuse animals. In 2019, the PACT Act (Preventing Animal Cruelty and Torture) finally made animal abuse a federal felony, although animal abusers still receive no mental health services upon conviction and animal abuse sentences tend to come with fairly mild punishments (Lee, 2019).

BSL causes challenges and suffering that social workers must be aware of and should seek to address. It keeps people out of housing, causes discrimination to disabled people with Pit Bull-type service dogs, limits accessible housing options, perpetrates institutionalized and systemic racism, and may cause extreme distress and trauma to the family if a dog is seized and destroyed (any discrimination toward service dogs due to BSL is a direct violation of the ADA, which does not discriminate against any breed of dog) (Lowrey, 2018). Taxpayer dollars are wasted on enforcing BSL with no basis in reality (a popular saying is "punish the deed, not the breed"). In December 2012, in an unprecedented initiative, the White House released a statement announcing that the Obama Administration stands firmly against breed-specific legislation (BSL) (Linder, 2018; Lowrey, 2018). Unfortunately, at the state and local levels, these laws continue to exist. It is important that clinical social workers are aware of the crisis that BSL can create for their clients, so that we may continue to advocate for them as best as we can.

Summary on Crisis Intervention for People with Pets

A person with pets may be in crisis in a number of ways that threaten not only the person's physical and material well-being, but their bond with their animal. Such crises include a lack of housing, food, or shelter; natural or man-made disasters; and domestic violence. The strictures of breed-specific legislation, meanwhile, may exacerbate or initiate crises for pet guardians, including jeopardizing access to housing. There are currently few studies on how the social determinants of health directly affect the well-being of humans, although research shows that pets help us live better lives (Johnson & Bruneau, 2019). Each time a practitioner is working on helping a client with concrete services, they have the opportunity to do clinical work; people in crisis are usually in a state of disequilibrium and require clinical interventions. It is important to keep in mind that people and their pets should be treated as a family unit, and that treating the person alone, without considering the needs of the family pet, will likely cause a rupture in the therapeutic alliance and prevent a client from fully healing. When we help people care for their pets we are caring for both the clinical and concrete needs of our clients. Some key questions to ask any client, to prepare for an emergency:

- Are you prepared to take your pets in an emergency?
- Do you have a disaster emergency kit?
- Would you evacuate without your pets?

Unfortunately, after the 9/11 terrorist attacks, many people were trapped uptown while their pets were trapped in the evacuation zone. This also caused undue hardship, as people who were already in crisis were caused more psychological trauma as the result of worrying about the needs of a pet that they were unable to access.

Some other questions to consider: What happens to pets when someone enters the hospital? What happens to pets when someone enters a psychiatric hospital?

What happens to pets when someone dies? People often forget to put their pets in their will or to speak to family about their wishes for their pets in case of emergency. Often it is assumed that the family will step up and care for the pet, although this is not always the case. Clinicians must keep in mind the many ways that clients with pets may be in crisis and the ways that we may advocate for the rights of our clients.

References

Abulof, U. (2017). Introduction: Why we need Maslow in the twenty-first century. *Society, 54*(6), 508–509.

Ascione, F. R. (2000). *Safe havens for pets: Guidelines for programs sheltering pets for women who are battered*. Available from http://www.vachss.com/guestdispatches/safe_havens.html

Baker, O. (2001). *A dog's life: Homeless people and their pets*. Blue Cross.

Banerjee, M. (2005). Applying Rawlsian justice to welfare reform. *Sociology & Social Welfare, 32*(3), 35–57.

Beetz, A., Uvnäs-Moberg, K., Julius, H., & Kotrschal, K. (2012). Psychosocial and psychophysiological effects of human-animal interactions: The possible role of oxytocin. *Frontiers in Psychology, 3*, 234.

Bender, K., Thompson, S. J., McManus, H., Lantry, J., & Flynn, P. M. (2007, February). Capacity for survival: Exploring strengths of homeless street youth. In *Child and youth care forum* (Vol. 36, No. 1, pp. 25–42). Kluwer Academic Publishers-Plenum Publishers.

Bulgakov, M. (2013). *The heart of a dog*. Melville House Pub.

Campbell, D. M. (2009). Pit bull bans: The state of breed-specific legislation. *GPSolo, 26*, 36.

Catala, A. (2015). Democracy, trust, and epistemic justice. *The Monist, 98*, 424–440.

Cohen, J., & Richardson, J. (2002). Pit bull panic. *Journal of Popular Culture, 36*(2), 285.

Compitus, K. (2019). Traumatic pet loss and the integration of attachment-based animal assisted therapy. *Journal of Psychotherapy Integration, 29*(2), 119.

Cronley, C., Strand, E. B., Patterson, D. A., & Gwaltney, S. (2009). Homeless people who are animal caretakers: A comparative study. *Psychological Reports, 105*(2), 481–499.

Dickey, B. (2017). *Pit bull: The battle over an American icon*. Vintages.

Duffy, D. L., Hsu, Y., & Serpell, J. A. (2008). Breed differences in canine aggression. *Applied Animal Behaviour Science, 114*(3-4), 441–460.

Edmonds, A. S., & Cutter, S. L. (2008). Planning for pet evacuations during disasters. *Journal of Homeland Security and Emergency Management, 5*(1), 1–18.

Graham, T. M. (2019). *Enhancing access to quality rental housing for people with pets as healthy public policy* (Unpublished doctoral thesis). University of Calgary. http://hdl.handle.net/1880/109854

Graham, T. M., Lucyk, K., Diep, L., & Rock, M. J. (2019). Discrimination towards people partnered with assistance dogs in Canada: Implications for policy and practice. *Society & Animals, 1*(aop), 1–36.

Gorant, J. (2011). *The lost dogs: Michael Vick's dogs and their tale of rescue and redemption*. Penguin.

Haden, S. C., McDonald, S. E., Booth, L. J., Ascione, F. R., & Blakelock, H. (2018). An exploratory study of domestic violence: Perpetrators' reports of violence against animals. *Anthrozoös, 31*(3), 337–352.

Hansen, S. (2020). *The impact of animal cruelty and future interpersonal violence: A quantitative study of disposed animal cruelty cases and criminal histories in Texas*. Doctoral dissertation, Northeastern University.

Howe, L., & Easterbrook, M. J. (2018). The perceived costs and benefits of pet ownership for homeless people in the UK: Practical costs, psychological benefits and vulnerability. *Journal of Poverty, 22*(6), 486–499.

Hunt, M., Al-Awadi, H., & Johnson, M. (2008). Psychological sequelae of pet loss following Hurricane Katrina. *Anthrozoös, 21*(2), 109–121.

Hutton, V. E. (2015). Social provisions of the human-animal relationship amongst 30 people living with HIV in Australia. *Anthrozoös, 28*(2), 199–214.

Irvine, L. (2013a). Animals as lifechangers and lifesavers: Pets in the redemption narratives of homeless people. *Journal of Contemporary Ethnography, 42*(1), 3–30.

Irvine, L. (2013b). *My dog always eats first: Homeless people and their animals*. Lynne Rienner Publishers.

Irvine, L. (2016). The person and the self as social accomplishment. *Animal Sentience, 1*(10), 11.

Irvine, L., Kahl, K. N., & Smith, J. M. (2012). Confrontations and donations: Encounters between homeless pet owners and the public. *The Sociological Quarterly, 53*(1), 25–43.

Johnson, A., & Bruneau, L. (2019). Pets and relationships: How animals help us understand ourselves and our connections with others. In *Clinician's guide to treating companion animal issues* (pp. 173–191). Academic Press.

Kidd, A. H., & Kidd, R. M. (1994). Benefits and liabilities of pets for the homeless. *Psychological Reports, 74*(3), 715–722.

Knight, S., & Edwards, V. (2008). In the company of wolves: the physical, social, and psychological benefits of dog ownership. *Journal of aging and health, 20*(4), 437–455.

Labrecque, J., & Walsh, C. A. (2011). Homeless women's voices on incorporating companion animals into shelter services. *Anthrozoös, 24*(1), 79–95.

LaVoy, E. (2019). The PETS Act and beyond: A critical examination of the PETS Act and what the future of disaster planning and response for animals should be. *Mitchell Hamline Law Journal of Public Policy & Practice, 40*, 67.

Ledger, R. A., Orihel, J. S., Clarke, N., Murphy, S., & Sedlbauer, M. (2005). Breed specific legislation: Considerations for evaluating its effectiveness and recommendations for alternatives. *The Canadian Veterinary Journal, 46*(8), 735.

Lee, C. G. (2019). *The PACT Act: A step in the right direction on the path to animal welfare*. Available at https://ssrn.com/abstract=3497003

Leonard, H. A., & Scammon, D. L. (2007). No pet left behind: Accommodating pets in emergency planning. *Journal of Public Policy & Marketing, 26*(1), 49–53.

Linder, A. (2018). The black man's dog: The social context of breed specific legislation. *Animal Law, 25*, 51.

Lockwood, R., & Rindy, K. (1987). Are "pit bulls" different? An analysis of the pit bull terrier controversy. *Anthrozoös, 1*(1), 2–8.

Lowrey, W. (2018). We the pit bulls: The fate of pit bulls under the United States constitution. *Animal Law, 24*, 373.

National Domestic Violence Hotline. (n.d.). Pet Safety During Domestic Violence. Retrieved from https://www.thehotline.org/plan-for-safety/pet-safety-during-domestic-violence/

Newberry, M. (2017). Pets in danger: Exploring the link between domestic violence and animal abuse. *Aggression and Violent Behavior, 34*, 273–281.

O'Haire, M. (2010). Companion animals and human health: Benefits, challenges, and the road ahead. *Journal of Veterinary Behavior, 5*(5), 226–234.

Olson, K. R., Levy, J. K., Norby, B., Crandall, M. M., Broadhurst, J. E., Jacks, S., Bartone, R. C., & Zimmerman, M. S. (2015). Inconsistent identification of pit bull-type dogs by shelter staff. *The Veterinary Journal, 206*(2), 197–202.

Parker, D. H. (2019, November). Proposal for robust person-to-person communications system for large-scale emergency displaced population of people and pets. In *2019 IEEE international symposium on technologies for homeland security (HST)* (pp. 1–8). IEEE.

Rew, L. (2000). Friends and pets as companions: Strategies for coping with loneliness among homeless youth. *Journal of Child and Adolescent Psychiatric Nursing, 13*(3), 125–132.

Rhoades, H., Winetrobe, H., & Rice, E. (2015). Pet ownership among homeless youth: Associations with mental health, service utilization and housing status. *Child Psychiatry & Human Development, 46*(2), 237–244.
Sen, A. (2004). Elements of a theory of human rights. *Philosophy and Public Affairs, 32*(4), 315.
Singer, R. S., Hart, L. A., & Zasloff, R. L. (1995). Dilemmas associated with rehousing homeless people who have companion animals. *Psychological Reports, 77*(3), 851–857.
Sobel, R. S., & Leeson, P. T. (2006). Government's response to Hurricane Katrina: A public choice analysis. *Public Choice, 127*(1-2), 55–73.
Stevenson, R., Fitzgerald, A., & Barrett, B. J. (2018). Keeping pets safe in the context of intimate partner violence: Insights from domestic violence shelter staff in Canada. *Affilia, 33*(2), 236–252.
Strand, E. B., & Faver, C. A. (2006). Battered women's concern for their pets: A closer look. *Journal of Family Social Work, 9*(4), 39–58.
Strauss, D., & Brulliard, K. (2018). Little by little, domestic violence shelters become pet friendly. *Washington Post*. Retrieved August, 2020 from https://www.washingtonpost.com/news/animalia/wp/2018/06/15/little-by-little-domestic-violence-shelters-become-pet-friendly/
Taylor, H., Williams, P., & Gray, D. (2004). Homelessness and dog ownership: An investigation into animal empathy, attachment, crime, drug use, health and public opinion. *Anthrozoös, 17*(4), 353–368.
United States. President of the United States, Assistant to the President for Homeland Security and Counterterrorism , Etats-Unis. Assistant to the President for homeland security and counterterrorism, Superintendent of Documents, Superintendent of Documents Staff. (2006). *The Federal Response to Hurricane Katrina: Lessons learned*. Government Printing Office.
U.S. Senate. Committee on Homeland Security and Governmental Affairs. (2006). *Hurricane Katrina: A nation still unprepared*. Government Printing Office. http://hsgac.senate.gov/_files/Katrina/FullReport.pdf
Vigdor, J. (2008). The economic aftermath of Hurricane Katrina. *Journal of Economic Perspectives, 22*(4), 135–154.
Walsh, F. (2009). Human-animal bonds II: The role of pets in family systems and family therapy. *Family Process, 48*(4), 481–499.
Wood, D. S., Weber, C. V., & Ascione, F. R. (1997). The abuse of animals and domestic violence: A national survey of shelters for women who are battered. *Society & Animals, 5*(3), 205–218.

Chapter 7
Current Research and Future Directions in the Human-Animal Bond

There are exciting research projects and programs currently being implemented in the human–animal bond (HAB) field. In this chapter, I will discuss some future directions of HAB research, and the clinical implications of HAB. These include the study of zooeyia, animal hoarding, and animal-assisted crisis intervention. These are all areas of study that appear very promising, but there is still a lack of research about each.

Zooeyia

"Zooeyia" is a term coined by researchers, taken from the Greek words for "animal" and "health" to describe the positive impact pet guardianship has on the health and well-being of human guardians (Hodgson & Darling, 2011). Pets benefit health by serving as builders of social capital, agents of harm reduction, and motivators for healthy behavioral change, and by being potential participants in their guardians' treatment plans (Hodgson et al., 2017). The development of a specific term for the benefits animals bestow is intended as a counterbalance to considerations related to zoonosis. Zoonosis is a word that describes the passing of a harmful disease from animals to humans; well-known zoonotic diseases include AIDS, SARS, and COVID-19. In fact, the vast majority (75%) of newly discovered diseases are actually zoonotic, which means they have originated in one species and have mutated enough to infect a host of a different species (such as humans) (Hodgson & Darling, 2011). However, zoonosis is not unidirectional and not limited to diseases; for example, zoonotic injuries include dog bites and cat scratches, while reverse zoonosis is the infection of other animal species with a disease that originated in humans. Hodgson and Darling (2011) explain that "zoonotic diseases emerging worldwide are due to multiple converging factors: climate change, increasing urbanization, human encroachment in wild areas, increased global travel and, for companion

K. Compitus, *The Human-Animal Bond in Clinical Social Work Practice*,
Essential Clinical Social Work Series,
https://doi.org/10.1007/978-3-030-87783-5_7

animals, increasing intimacy with humans" (p. 189). There is extensive research done in the field of zoonosis, which is why Hodgson and Darling (2011) created the word "Zooeyia" as the "positive inverse of zoonosis" in order to describe the numerous benefits that result from interaction between humans and other species of animals. These benefits include the biological/physiological, the psychological, and the social welfare-related, and apply to both humans and their pets. In essence, zooeyia may be viewed as the human–animal bond as seen through a biopsychosocial framework.

Hodgson and Darling's concept came from a paper that emerged from the One Health movement. The CDC administers the One Health program and defines it as "a collaborative, multisectoral, and transdisciplinary approach—working at the local, regional, national, and global levels—with the goal of achieving optimal health outcomes recognizing the interconnection between people, animals, plants, and their shared environment" (CDC, 2021). The movement is founded on the understanding that humans and their pets living in close proximity results in a reciprocal effect on the health and well-being of both (Natterson-Horowitz & Bowers, 2012). In the One Health program, pets and their people are not considered in isolation, but within the context of how the health of one affects the health of the other. For example, many medical conditions are seen both in humans and other species of animals, such as cancer or cardiomyopathy (Natterson-Horowitz & Bowers, 2012). When human doctors treat the people in isolation, they don't consider the health benefits that the interaction effect provides. As discussed previously, these benefits can include an increase in physical activity, a decrease in anxiety or depression, an increase in social interaction, an increased sense of safety, or even the elimination or prevention of substance abuse.

One Health promotes the benefits of integrating human and animal medicine (Gibbs, 2014) to heal both participants. For example, we can learn more about the sources of some diseases, such as cancer, by studying how it evolves in other species. Yet, to date, human doctors rarely consider veterinary medicine in their research or diagnostic assessment, while veterinarians (who are taught to treat more than one species of animal) often look across species for clues to diagnosis and treatment. One Health considers that both human medical doctors and veterinarians have much to learn from each other and can benefit from working together; its proponents suggest that health facilities should have both types of doctors working in conjunction in the same clinic. Although it seems a little different from how we normally treat illnesses, there may be many benefits to people if they are able to schedule veterinary appointments at the same time and place as their own medical appointments (this could especially benefit vulnerable populations with limited resources such as those who are homeless, seniors with mobility issues, and the parents of young children, among others).

As discussed earlier, studies suggest pet guardianship has a number of health benefits, with implications at the societal level in terms of healthcare costs. Research evidence from Germany and Australia show pet guardians have improvement in chronic illness symptoms, and therefore fewer doctor visits than their non-pet guardian counterparts. These effects created an estimated savings of over 5.59

million euros in Germany and 3.86 billion Australian dollars annually (Headey et al., 2002). If treating human medical patients through an HAB lens with a biopsychosocial framework not only saves money but potentially improves the welfare of pets and their people, then it is a program that warrants further attention and research.

The social determinants of health are the conditions in the environment in which people are born and live that affect a wide range of health and quality-of-life outcomes (and risks). These conditions (social, economic, physical) in various settings (school, home, work) determine people's sense of engagement and security where they live. Resources that enhance these conditions may have a significant influence on a person's quality of life and public health outcomes. Unpublished data obtained through social determinants of health screenings in the Montefiore Medical Group since 2018 shows that out of 41,611 screens during the period, 7602 individuals endorsed at least one social determinant of health factor. Of those reporting social determinants of health issues, 1873 reported healthcare transportation difficulties, 1484 reported difficulty paying healthcare costs, 2271 reported financial insecurity, and 2392 reported issues of housing quality. Each of these factors may be affected by pet ownership; for example, pet owners may face financial burdens or housing challenges related to their pets. Therefore, rather than simply celebrating zooeyia as a "free bonus" that improves health outcomes, public health discussions should consider how pet guardianship can be facilitated and its burdens eased with regard to social determinants of health. For example, choosing to remain non-domiciled secondary to a shelter's refusal to admit the animal may cause distress to both the person and their pet (Rhoades et al., 2015). Research into the social determinants of health as they affect pet guardians is, therefore, an area that warrants further study.

Animal Hoarding

I am often asked about the difference between an animal sanctuary and animal hoarding, and it boils down to the well-being and care of all involved. Sanctuary owners may have large numbers of animals, but they get frequent medical care for the animals and maintain a consistently clean environment for the animals. Animal hoarders believe that they are saving the animals but are unable to provide responsible care once the animal has entered their home.

Despite having distinct properties, animal hoarding is not currently a separate category from item hoarding in the *Diagnostic and Statistical Manual of Mental Disorders* (DSM-5). Hoarding Disorder (item hoarding) is characterized as a persistent difficulty discarding possessions, regardless of their actual value (Mataix-Cols et al., 2010). The person who is hoarding feels a strong need to save the items and feels extreme distress when presented with the idea of discarding these items. As a result, hoarders accumulate a large number of items that clutter and congest their living areas, potentially compromising their own health and safety (Kalogeraki & Michopoulos, 2017).

Animal hoarders, like item hoarders, tend to amass a large number of animals and feel unable to give them away. According to Ferreira et al. (2017), only about 56% of animal hoarders also hoard nonliving items. The average age of an animal hoarder is 61 years old and the vast majority (73%) are women (Ferreira et al., 2017). The average number of animals in an animal hoarding situation was approximately 41. Unlike hoarded objects, hoarded animals do not usually obstruct environments, although they will often live in such disarray that the authorities may be called to the house because of the smells or noises from the animals. Usually the hoarders fail to provide the animals with a basic standard of nutrition, sanitation, and veterinary care, and studies show that many animals suffer greatly or die painfully in these houses (Frost et al., 2011).

Animal hoarding is distinct from item hoarding because of the emotional aspect of the human-animal bond. The motivation behind animal hoarding is different; the hoarders often think that they are saving or helping animals in need. However, animal hoarders are usually unable to see that they are misjudging the best interests of the animal, and the hoarders usually have little to no insight into their condition. Animal hoarding, like item hoarding, happens gradually over time and usually after a traumatic incident (often the death of a loved one) that causes the hoarder to want to make an emotional connection to another living being in order to fill the void. Most hoarders in one study had had large numbers of animals for at least 23 years before receiving intervention services (Ferreira, 2017) and, as stated above, intervention only happens when the situation becomes so dire that the authorities are called. Unfortunately, lacking insight into their condition, animal hoarders often do not want to accept help and animal hoarding is sometimes characterized as a type of delusional disorder. Most often, local animal control services have to forcibly remove the animals from the person's home.

The removal of the animals is to help the suffering animals but also to help the person, since the house may be so filthy—filled with feces, urine, dead animals, bugs, and rodents—that the person's health will suffer as much as the animals. Sadly, the forcible removal of the animals does nothing to treat the mental disorder of the hoarder and the recidivism rate is high in animal hoarding cases (Frost et al., 2011). There are few mental health agencies or clinicians that specialize in animal hoarding, which means that usually intervention services target only the neglected animals. Since the person does not receive mental health treatment, and has no insight into their condition, there is nothing to prevent the person from acquiring new animals soon after local authorities remove the existing neglected animals.

It is estimated that there are 700–2000 new cases of animal hoarding in the United States each year (Frost et al., 2011). Unlike in item hoarding, which often starts in childhood, animal hoarding often happens in late middle age (Frost et al., 2011). Animal hoarders tend to hoard only one species of animal (most frequently dogs or cats) (and researchers hypothesize that approximately 31% of animal hoarders will also hoard other items), while item hoarders may collect a large variety of types of items (paper, newspapers, clothes, containers, etc.) (Frost et al., 2011). Another difference is that animal hoarders may obtain their animals through either active or passive means—by either adopting or rescuing the animals, or by failing to spay/neuter existing animals and allowing them to quickly multiply. The Hoarding of Animals Research Consortium (HARC) suggests that animal hoarding is likely a delusional disorder and has characteristics similar to those of attachment-related disorders (Frost, 2000). The people who hoard animals report a strong sense of emotional attachment to their animals and will often choose relationships with their animals over connecting with family members. Consistent with a delusional disorder, many animal hoarders believe that they have special magical powers or a special ability that allows them to communicate with animals (Frost et al., 2011).

Since animal hoarders often do not receive intervention services until the authorities are called, they often find themselves with legal problems. There can be eviction notices, health code violations, or the home may be condemned as unsafe. In addition, animal hoarders may find themselves charged with criminal cruelty to animals and in some states hoarding itself is a criminal offence (Frost et al., 2011).

If animal hoarding is a mental disorder, how can we help treat animal hoarders to reduce the rates of recidivism? Mental health practitioners must get involved in the direct treatment of animal hoarders. The hoarder should receive mental health treatment as needed, including grief counseling, a strong therapeutic alliance, and counseling aimed at reducing social isolation and forming or strengthening emotional attachments to other humans (Patronek & Nathanson, 2009). Agencies that address animal hoarding should collaborate, including animal rescue agencies, local law enforcement, health departments, veterinarians, and social service agencies, since there are multiple victims involved (including the hoarder themselves) (Reinisch, 2008). Since the hoarders have a strong attachment to the animals in their care, to remove the animals may cause another traumatic attachment rupture; it is recommended that, although the majority of the animals in the house should be removed, the hoarder should be allowed to keep some of the animals, after they have received proper veterinary medical treatment (vaccinations, spay/neutering). Early intervention is key to helping animal hoarders and the animals in their care. Therefore, we need more research to help identify risk factors as well as more intervention services and more access to mental health treatment for people suffering from an animal hoarding disorder.

Animal-Assisted Crisis Response (AACR)

The dangers in our world are many, from terrorist attacks and school shootings to natural disasters such as tsunamis, earthquakes, and hurricanes. These types of horrifying events throw people into a state of crisis. Mental health first responders must use their crisis intervention skills to help the people affected by these tragedies return to a state of equilibrium. This can be a very difficult task, and the rate of burnout for crisis intervention workers is often high. Crisis intervention mental health workers frequently work as a team to help alleviate this burden, and sometimes animals are a part of that team. For over 30 years, animals have been used as members of crisis response teams, demonstrating the power of the human–animal bond as an often overlooked relationship that can be utilized by mental health professionals to strengthen and support the ego functioning of individuals in crisis. The animals not only provide comfort and hope for those affected by crisis and disasters, but they also help create a faster rapport between those affected by the crisis and mental health first responders. Although animal-assisted crisis response is well established over several decades, there is little information about the efficacy of therapy animals as crisis first responders. With the number of natural and man-made disasters on the rise, it is important to have effective crisis intervention treatment options.

AACR Model

Animal attachment can be used not only during formal therapy, but also during disaster relief efforts to increase resilience (Thompson et al., 2014). Animal-Assisted Crisis Response utilizes therapy animals to provide comfort, support, and a sense of safety for trauma, crisis, and disaster survivors. It has traditionally involved "Animal-Assisted Activities," a third type of intervention. The International Association for Human–Animal Interaction Organizations defines Animal-Assisted Activity (AAA) as:

> *informal interactions/visitations often conducted on a volunteer basis by the human-animal team for motivational, educational and recreational purposes. There are no treatment goals for the interactions. AAAs are generally facilitated by individuals who do not have a health, education or human service degree. Human-animal teams have received at least introductory training, preparation and assessment to participate in informal visitations.* (IAHAIO, 2014)

This can include visits to nursing homes, schools, and other facilities with the primary purpose of bringing pleasure and comfort to the clients without any intended therapeutic outcome. This is how Animal-Assisted Crisis Relief started.

AACR teams respond directly to major disasters with therapy dogs and their handlers to provide therapeutic aid to trauma survivors. The first major AACR disaster response was the Oklahoma City bombing in 1995. The federal government requested that a newly formed organization, Therapy Dogs International, respond to the crisis by bringing therapy dogs to the scene to provide comfort not only to the victims and their families but also to the first responders (Shubert, 2012). In 1998, Therapy Dogs International (TDI) responded to the shooting at Thurston High School at the request of the National Organization for Victims' Assistance (Shubert, 2012). Another AACR organization, HOPE, was soon formed and was contacted by the American Red Cross to travel to New York City to provide animal-assisted crisis intervention in response to the September 11, 2001 terrorist attack on the World Trade Center (Shubert, 2012). The animal and handler teams spent two weeks of multiple shifts throughout each day at Ground Zero (always keeping the welfare of the animals in mind). Since the handlers are usually not trained mental health professionals, they were paired with mental health professionals for the duration of the crisis intervention. The mental health crisis intervention workers later wrote in detail about the benefit of having therapy animals on site, stating "the presence of the dogs had allowed them to connect with the recovery workers in ways that would have been very difficult if they had been alone" (Shubert, 2012, p. 75).

There are a number of ways that therapy animals can be beneficial to a mental health crisis intervention worker. The animals provide a therapeutic bridge and help the psychotherapists to engage and establish a rapport with the survivors and first responders. Cindy Ehlers is the founder of the HOPE Pets program within the Delta Society and she also developed the first special crisis response training for pet partner teams (Shubert, 2012). Shubert (2012) wrote that:

> *The animals served as symbols of qualities that individuals had or wished they had (i.e.,, afraid, helpless, brave, strong) or they were used to communicate thoughts and feelings indirectly (i.e., speaking for the dog: "she's afraid"). [Ehlers] pointed out that the animals helped to normalize the situation for the responders by reminding them of their lives outside of the situation. In addition, petting the animals is known to exert a calming effect by facilitating the body's production of oxytocin, a hormone known to produce a calming effect. These effects were noticeable to the human members of the teams. Last, the animals served as protective shields for the families riding the ferry boats to view Ground Zero and enabled them to begin to find the strength to deal with their losses.* (Shubert, 2012, p. 75)

There were approximately 500 animal and handler teams that responded to the September 11 terrorist attacks, consisting of dogs of all breeds and sizes, as well as some cats. Perhaps one of the reasons that animals are so efficient in helping people in crisis return to a state of equilibrium is that they often serve as a transitional object, orienting people by providing a reality-based relationship that comforts by alleviating physiological and psychological stress. The animals may provide a grounding experience and a way to encourage reality testing by helping survivors and first responders acknowledge that, although the current situation is life-changing, they will eventually be able to return to a state of normality and begin to heal.

Since the establishment of TDI and HOPE, the organizations have responded to numerous crisis events, including Hurricanes Katrina, Rita, and Ike; multiple school and university shootings; and the tenth memorial of September 11 (Shubert, 2012). Therapy dogs, and even therapy miniature horses, were brought in to Sandy Hook Elementary School after the tragic shooting there. AACR is thought to be highly effective in returning people in crisis to a state of emotional equilibrium, though it remains an animal-assisted activity rather than animal-assisted therapy unless the handler and animal are specifically paired with mental health professionals, as they were at the World Trade Center site.

Kelly (2017) believes that "the informal nature of these types of activities contrasts them with the goal-oriented nature of AAT, in which the therapy program is customized around the needs of individual patients or the needs associated with a particular treatment or condition" (p. 422). I have to disagree with that assessment. Crisis intervention is a particular short-term intervention that is designed around the needs of survivors and first-responders. It may be less structured than therapy, but it certainly is goal-oriented. Kelly explains that people in crisis often feel a lack of control over their immediate environment and, as such, may benefit from observing the positive and trusting relationship between the therapist and therapy animal (Kelly & Cozzolino, 2015). Although the handlers of AACR are not trained mental health professionals, they certainly do model this positive relationship. Rogers & Soyka (2004) states that the presence of therapy animals at a crisis site allowed first responders to "connect with workers in ways that would have been much more difficult if the dogs had not paved the way." The animals facilitate a relationship between the mental health professional and the client that expedites the therapeutic response. People in crisis may be in shock and may forget how to interact with other people; at such times, the animal will serve as a bridge back to interpersonal connections. Finally, since they cannot dwell on the past but are living in the moment, the dogs may symbolize hope to many (Thompson et al., 2014).

Perhaps there should be more licensed mental health professionals paired with AACR teams and, in this way, we will not only provide comfort to those in crisis but can also provide formal short-term AAT to those in need. To date, a large number of AACR teams have responded to disasters and provided relief to thousands of people. An attachment to animals can clearly be used to increase resilience in survivors and first responders. It is certainly a phenomenon worth further study.

Clinical Implications

The human–animal bond is a large and burgeoning field that requires additional research and development. When we examine the HAB, we note that the well-being of people and animals are often so closely intertwined that to address the needs of one is to improve the welfare of both. Since the HAB remains undervalued across the board, the gaps in services involving people with pets in crisis are many, and must be addressed.

There is some speculation that "extremely weak or strong HABs may be correlated with a reduced capacity to build resilience and process adversity" (Hill et al., 2020). This warrants further study so that we can better understand what may be a complex relationship between HAB and resilience. In any case, we should consider the HAB when helping our clients build resilience, whether through AAT, disaster relief services, or when working with animal hoarders. There appears to also be a strong connection between HAB and perceived social support (from other humans) (Hill et al., 2020), and animals should be regarded for their capacity as a social lubricant to help people connect to each other (Wood et al., 2015).

There are a variety of ways in which animals may influence our lives. It is time to include HAB in our clinical choices and include questions about pets on mental health intake forms. The more we know about how people connect to their pets, the better we may be able to help them connect to the rest of the world.

References

Centers for Disease Control and Prevention (CDC). (2021). *One health*. Retrieved from https://www.cdc.gov/onehealth/index.html

Ferreira, E. A., Paloski, L. H., Costa, D. B., Fiametti, V. S., De Oliveira, C. R., de Lima Argimon, I. I., Gonzatti, V., & Irigaray, T. Q. (2017). Animal hoarding disorder: A new psychopathology? *Psychiatry Research, 258*, 221–225.

Frost, R. (2000). People who hoard animals. *Psychiatric Times, 17*(4), 367–382.

Frost, R. O., Patronek, G., & Rosenfield, E. (2011). Comparison of object and animal hoarding. *Depression and Anxiety, 28*(10), 885–891.

Gibbs, E. P. J. (2014). The evolution of one health: A decade of progress and challenges for the future. *Veterinary Record, 174*(4), 85–91.

Headey, B., Grabka, M., Kelley, J., Reddy, P., & Tseng, Y. P. (2002). Pet ownership is good for your health and saves public expenditure too: Australian and German longitudinal evidence. *Australian Social Monitor, 5*(4), 93–99.

Hill, L., Winefield, H., & Bennett, P. (2020). Are stronger bonds better? Examining the relationship between the human–animal bond and human social support, and its impact on resilience. *Australian Psychologist, 55*(6), 729–738.

Hodgson, K., & Darling, M. (2011). Zooeyia: An essential component of "One Health". *The Canadian Veterinary Journal, 52*(2), 189.

Hodgson, K., Darling, M., Freeman, D., & Monavvari, A. (2017). Asking about pets enhances patient communication and care: a pilot study. *INQUIRY: The Journal of Health Care Organization, Provision, and Financing, 54*, 0046958017734030.

International Association of Human-Animal Interaction Organizations. (2014). *White paper on animal-assisted interventions*. Retrieved March 4, 2018, from http://iahaio.org/best-practice/white-paper-on-animal-assisted-interventions/

Kalogeraki, L., & Michopoulos, I. (2017). Hoarding disorder in DSM-5: Clinical description and cognitive approach. *Psychiatrike= Psychiatriki, 28*(2), 131–141.

Kelly, M. A., & Cozzolino, C. A. (2015). Helping at-risk youth overcome trauma and substance abuse through animal-assisted therapy. *Contemporary Justice Review, 18*(4), 421–434.

Mataix-Cols, D., Frost, R. O., Pertusa, A., Clark, L. A., Saxena, S., Leckman, J. F., Stein, D. J., Matsunaga, H., & Wilhelm, S. (2010). Hoarding disorder: A new diagnosis for DSM-V? *Depression and Anxiety, 27*(6), 556–572.

Natterson-Horowitz, B., & Bowers, K. (2012). *Zoobiquity: What animals can teach us about health and the science of healing*. Vintage.

Patronek, G. J., & Nathanson, J. N. (2009). A theoretical perspective to inform assessment and treatment strategies for animal hoarders. *Clinical Psychology Review, 29*(3), 274–281.

Reinisch, A. I. (2008). Understanding the human aspects of animal hoarding. *The Canadian Veterinary Journal, 49*(12), 1211.

Rogers, J. R., & Soyka, K. M. (2004). "One size fits all": An existential-constructivist perspective on the crisis intervention approach with suicidal individuals. *Journal of Contemporary Psychotherapy, 34*(1), 7–22.

Shubert, J. (2012). Therapy dogs and stress management assistance during disasters. *U.S. Army Medical Department Journal, 4*, 74–78.

Thompson, K., Every, D., Rainbird, S., Cornell, V., Smith, B., & Trigg, J. (2014). No pet or their person left behind: Increasing the disaster resilience of vulnerable groups through animal attachment, activities and networks. *Animals (2076–2615), 4*(2), 214–240.

Wood, L., Martin, K., Christian, H., Nathan, A., Lauritsen, C., Houghton, S., Kawachi, I., & McCune, S. (2015). The pet factor-companion animals as a conduit for getting to know people, friendship formation and social support. *PLoS One, 10*(4), e0122085.

Index

K. Compitus, *The Human-Animal Bond in Clinical Social Work Practice*, Essential Clinical Social Work Series,
https://doi.org/10.1007/978-3-030-87783-5

GPSR Compliance
The European Union's (EU) General Product Safety Regulation (GPSR) is a set of rules that requires consumer products to be safe and our obligations to ensure this.

If you have any concerns about our products, you can contact us on

ProductSafety@springernature.com

In case Publisher is established outside the EU, the EU authorized representative is:

Springer Nature Customer Service Center GmbH
Europaplatz 3
69115 Heidelberg, Germany

www.ingramcontent.com/pod-product-compliance
Lightning Source LLC
Chambersburg PA
CBHW052139150725
29676CB00003B/115
* 9 7 8 3 0 3 0 8 7 7 8 2 8 *